GW01090534

Healthy Bunch CookBook

Trisha Stewart

Healthy Bunch Cook Book

The Essential Vegan Cook Book for all you Healthy Tarts, Healthy Dudes and Healthy Idols. Fabulous recipes to create delicious meals while optimizing your weight and health!

By Trisha Stewart

Healthy Bunch Cook Book

Visit us on the web at:
www.TrishaStewart.com
www.HealthyBunchCookBook.com
www.HealthyTart.com
www.HealthyDudeBook.com
www.HealthyIdol.com

ISBN 978-0-9816846-3-5

Other books by Trisha Stewart include:
      Healthy Tart
      Healthy Idol
      Healthy Dude Book

Books by Christin McDowell
      Healthy Fitness Central

Trisha Stewart

Dedications

To All You Wannabe Healthy Tart's, Dude's and Idols

Nothing will benefit human health and increase the chances for survival of life on Earth as much as the evolution to a vegetarian diet.

Albert Einstein

Trisha Stewart

Contents

Introduction

This cookery book has been created to support the series of books I have already written on diet and lifestyle - Healthy Tart - Healthy Idol - Healthy Dude and (Healthy Fitness Central which is written by my great friend and colleague, and our own fitness guru Christin McDowell). Healthy Pumpkin will be in print by the early 2009 with more to follow.

The Healthy Bunch Cookbook is deliberately focusing on vegetarian/vegan foods to support these great lifestyle books, but also to encourage those people who eat flesh and dairy to try some great alternatives. Even though I have outlined in my other books very good reasons to avoid eating animal produce I know some people will continue to do so; which is all about choices. Choosing recipes in this book will greatly contribute to your own health and wellness and that of your family and friends. You will be amazed how many people love to eat this kind of food. Help to spread the word about a great way of eating for optimum health and make this book part of your everyday eating regime.

I have deliberately not used any fake, commercially produced cheeze, bacon bits, chicken this or that; everything you are going to produce from this book will be made entirely from your own raw ingredients... that way you know exactly what will be in each recipe.

What could be better than sampling your own fresh cooked or raw meals, from ingredients you have grown, swapped with a neighbor, bought from the local farmers market and picked from the hedgerow, even from your hanging basket; ever put Nasturtiums in a salad ? The flowers and leaves are edible and make such a lovely display.

The window ledge in your house, conservatory or greenhouse is perfect for growing herbs and some vegetables or fruits such as tomatoes, chillies and aubergine/eggplant; they will produce small but really tasty produce to add to your raw meals or your cooked meals, depending on the time of year.

The recipes are a mix of cultures but with no wheat, dairy, sugar (refined) or yeast - the food will not be boring, I promise you. The meals are all packed with fresh flavor and color. They are very nutritious and suitable for the whole family; no matter what their age.

Meals packed full of fiber, carbohydrates (slow release for lots of long term energy), protein, essential fats (very little saturated, only from coconut), vitamins, minerals, enzymes and bioflavanoids.

I have even included a chapter on how to pack a lunch box for your whole family, full of fabulous food to eat on the go, no need to stop off at any junk food takeaway or grab something from the office or school vending machine.

Imagine those glossy red peppers and purple aubergines/eggplants, fat onions and fennel bulbs, cloves of garlic and fresh ginger root, bright green spinach and curly kale, vibrant orange carrots and deep purple beetroot/beets - get those digestive juices flowing, smell the herbs, fresh basil, parsley, tarragon, thyme, sage - just to name a few that you are going to add to your luscious food! Mmmmm........

Taste the lovely oils, olive, sesame, sunflower and coconut. Take in the aroma of the spices, cumin, coriander, turmeric, garam masala and start to blend all of this in your mind. I am going to show you how to put it all together; you just need to keep thinking about these wonderful foods.

Beans, kidney, flageolet, haricot, mung, adzuki with lentils, wholegrain rice, quinoa, millet and buckwheat; all these can be cooked into fabulous stews and casseroles, curries and chillies... you can even sprout them and eat raw.

Spread nut and seed butters onto fresh baked oatcakes, make vegan cheeze, mayo and other dips and marinades, Instead of sugar or commercial sweeteners I have used natural fruits, pure maple syrup and honey (for non Vegan's); be indulgent in foods that will not harm you... only help to heal you and keep you full of that health and vitality I am always going on about.

Choose homemade muesli and make a lovely porridge for breakfast, not just the hum drum ready cereals you are used to; cook quick dinners or snacks, make all your own curry paste and sauces, no more jars of this stuff for you.

I want everyone to become excited about eating real whole foods and this book is the first in a series of cooking and non cooking books. Yes, I will be bringing you some more fabulous recipes and menu ideas for raw foods and not just salads! But with the emphasis on eating with the seasons as I believe that eating according to what is in season is what we are designed to do. Warm in winter, cool in the summer. Of course if your climate is warm all the time then you have a really wide choice of foods all year round.

I would also like you to think about "air miles." How far does your food have to travel before it gets to your table? Less is best, so buy as local as possible.

Having worked with a wide range of clients, some of who have never cooked anything from base ingredients and who think a meal comes in a box from the supermarket or takeaway, to those who really know their way around a kitchen. I am continually being asked for ways to create interesting but quick whole foods, so this book is going to show you just that. There are also some recipes that take a while to prepare and cook but I do feel that spending time in the kitchen is very rewarding;

the creation of a meal for yourself or others should really feature in your life as it is nourishing for the body and soul.

There are 'quick to make' desserts and puddings, and ice creams using only healthy ingredients; you will never buy a commercial product again after tasting your own home made. A range of dips, dressings, pate's and sauces, cream and cheeze which can all be made up in a few minutes; soups, curries, stuffed vegetables, salads, desserts, bean cuisine and all sorts to tempt everyone's palate. This book has been deliberately created so that you can use core base ingredients for a variety of dishes to save time.

Every recipe has a "tip" or more than one "tip". These tips serve to expand the recipe rather than write five different recipes on how to make a curry, chilli or whatever. For instance, stuffing vegetables is easy; a base recipe with varying ingredients can be made into several different meals or snacks. So, whilst this book does not have hundreds of pages, it is absolutely packed with easy to use recipes that will make many different meals. Make sure you check out those "tips" to tailor your own recipes.

Time – one of the main obstacles many people face. Whilst some of the recipes will take more time than others, there are some quick meals for when you just get in from work or for when friends turn up and are hungry; or everyone is due out of the house in 1 hour and has to eat.

Planning ahead is the key to a healthy kitchen, there are foods you can cook in advance, keep refrigerated or freeze so that you always have some basic ingredients ready on hand. Also, learn how to create your own deli in the refrigerator, including really healthy sprouts. The kids will love these and could be in charge of the growing and harvesting of them, just watch their faces as these sprouts grow in super fast time – fantastically healthy and quick.

There are explanations to all the ingredients that feature in the book, a lot of these will be store cupboard goods that will keep for 6 months; others will be fresh, growing in the window box or garden or available at your local farmers market.

Check out the information on the main food groups, what they do and why we need them. Not too much reading here though as there is a full resource on www.trishastewart.com

Some tips on kitchen equipment that you will need to make life easy, chances are if you have read Healthy Tart you will know all about this. If not, there is a quick reminder in this book.

All the lovely ingredients in this book will contribute to fabulous good health. I have deliberately refrained from adding food values as by eating this type of food you don't need to worry whether you are having too much saturated fat or too much sugar. This way of eating is always going to be healthy and does not contain those foods that will contribute to ill health, heart disease, cancer or diabetes. You can of course eat too much of a good thing so beware of overeating any foods; equally not eating enough can be a problem. There is more about that on my website and in the other 'Healthy Lifestyle' books.

I would also like to encourage you to work with your senses, your eyes and nose; working with a variety of herbs and spices, let your nose do the work for you, smell what you are going to put into your food, see if it works for you... there are no hard and fast rules about what herb or spice goes with anything - we are all about choices so use those senses. Create colorful meals that smell good and you will have everyone demanding food!

This is not just another cookbook and it is definitely not another diet book, this is a book dedicated to those who want to be healthy, have fun with food and enjoy their lives to the full.

Being full of health and vitality has to be the best way to live your life and if you have been reading my other books Healthy Tart, Healthy Idol and Healthy Dude Book you will note that all of my books are re-educating you into living your best life ever.

You will never want to go back to eating from a supermarket shelf, diner or takeaway joint – if you do you will be very disappointed at the taste of it, salty, tasteless, full of chemicals and so on...here I go again on my soapbox!

If you are diabetic or have candida then I would advise you to omit the sweetened recipes. If you are concerned about any of the recipes and your health, please go to my 24/7 online resource www.trishastewart.com and check in with me to make sure you are doing all the right things.

I have included a shopping list, not complete as you will need to decide what fresh ingredients you are going to use, but all the store cupboard necessities are listed. Refer to the back of the book as it briefly explains the ingredients we are using and their benefits.

Okay, so let's rock and roll into the kitchen, dive out to the farmers market and get going on the highway to health. What are you waiting for?

Bon appetite!

Great Start to the Day

Breakfast really is important. The recipes in this section are designed to help you stave of hunger till lunchtime. However, you can choose anything you like for breakfast, so don't be tied to this section – maybe you would enjoy a soup for breakfast, I do, especially in

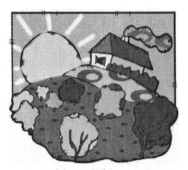

winter in the UK, or a juice or a smoothie. Whatever you choose from this book will be packed full of nutritious ingredients to have at any time of the day.

Healthy Bunch Porridge

Per person (large portion to keep you going all morning)

- A cupful of oats to 2 cups of water or a mix of water and non dairy milk
- Put in a small pan, just bring to simmer for a few minutes, add more fluid if mixture is too dry.
- Or/ just pour boiling water over the dry oats and allow to soak for 5 minutes (that's my favorite way as it is quick and easy and you don't get a dirty pan!)

Tips

Add any of the following:

- Pure vanilla essence or a vanilla pod

- Nutmeg
- Cinnamon
- Nuts and Seeds, ground or whole
- Fresh stewed fruit
- A little soy yogurt
- A little cream (see recipes for dairy alternatives)
- Try another grain such as millet or quinoa or a mix of all three

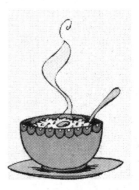

Healthy Bunch Muesli

Per person (large portion to keep you going all morning)

- ¼ cup each of rice flakes, oats and millet flakes
- Add chopped nuts, sunflower seeds, sesame seeds, pumpkin seeds and flax seed
- Soak in soy or rice milk, apple or other juice, for half an hour or less -if you like the mixture a little dry
- Top with fresh fruit and/or cream (see recipes for dairy alternatives)

Tips

- Make up a batch of the dry ingredients and keep in an airtight container

Healthy Bunch Granola

Enough for four good sized servings

(Be aware! this is delicious but covered in calories! Take a little at a time; I recommend sprinkling a small handful on top of porridge or fresh fruit rather than having a full portion)

115g/4oz/1cup	Each of porridge oats, jumbo oats
50g/2oz/ ½ cup	Each of sesame and sunflower seeds
50g/2oz/ ½ cup	Hazelnuts
25g/1oz/ ¼ cup	Almonds coarsely chopped
50ml/2fl oz/ ¼ cup	Sunflower oil
50ml/2fl oz/ ¼ cup	Honey or if vegan, maple syrup

Directions

- Heat oven to 140c/275f/gas 1
- Put the oil and honey/maple syrup into a pan and gently warm through to get a runny consistency. Remove from heat
- Add the rest of the ingredients, mix well
- Turn out onto one or more baking sheets, make sure the ingredients are spread well so they can all toast and not stick together
- Bake for around 45-50mins, you may need to stir or shake to separate the ingredients
- Remove from the oven and allow to cool completely
- Put into an airtight container

Tips

- These will keep for a few weeks, if no one eats it all straight away! so if you want more double up the quantities and store in an airtight container.

Buckwheat Pancakes

Will make around 4-6 pancakes, depending on size of pan

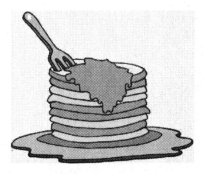

This is a basic recipe; you may like to play around with different ingredients to make this work for you. They will not be as light as the usual pancakes as you are using a different kind of flour.

115g/4oz/1 cup	Buckwheat flour
2 tsp	Baking powder
Pinch	Sea salt
8floz/1 cup	Soy milk, rice milk or almond milk
1 tsp	pure vanilla essence
2 tbsp	Ground almonds or finely chopped walnuts

Preparation

- Mix all the ingredients in a bowl with a whisk or put into a blender

- Heat a little coconut or olive oil in a pan and ladle in the mixture to cover the base of the pan. Cook for a minute or so on each side.

Tips

- Fill each pancake with some lovely fresh fruit or some stewed fruits and top with a little cream (see recipes) or a savory such as wilted spinach with nutmeg

---

Tofu Scramble

---

4 servings

1 pack	Tofu (softer variety or silken is best)
1	Small onion finely diced
1	Clove diced garlic
4 tbsp	Red pepper, courgette/zucchini, whatever you have diced
Pinch	Turmeric or cumin or other spices or herbs that you like
1 tbsp	Olive oil or coconut oil to fry in

Preparation

- Drain and crumble the Tofu
- Sauté off the onion, garlic, spices or herbs (if fresh leave herbs till last)
- Add tofu and your choice of vegetables, cook till they are to your liking

Tips

This a simple recipe, packed with protein. Try a variation of vegetables or use some raw sprouts for a change.

Fresh Fruit Salads

How many ways can you make a fresh fruit salad – well quite simple, as many as you like but please choose organic fruits with the least amount of air or road miles on them, that makes eating in season a good thing, although your choices may be limited at times you will definitely be eating some of the

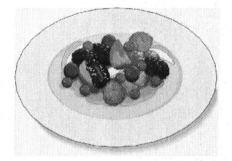

best and naturally ripened fruits if you choose local produce.

Take anything from juicy oranges to crunchy apples. Try a feast of raspberries, strawberries, blackberries, blueberries; Plump plums, cherries, fresh figs and apricots. Try exotic mango and papaya, pomegranates, star fruit. Watery fruits such as melon and cantaloupe, to fruits such as grapes, pears, kiwi, guava and banana. The citrus family, clementine, satsuma, mineola, tangerine, grapefruits, limes, lemons and kumquat. Try lots of scrummy fruits, tons of flavor and color, loads of enzymes and other nutrients.

Preparation of fruits

- Wash or rinse
- Peel those that have to be peeled

- Cut into eatable sizes, or slice, cube whatever works best
- If you need to make a fruit salad liquid, squeeze some oranges or press apples or blend some berries.

Here are some ideas on how to make sure you display your lovely fruits

- One of the key ingredients is choosing a lovely dish
- For one serving take a nice large pretty dish
- If you are serving your family or friends choose from a large bowl to a shallow platter
- Cut a pineapple in half, carefully cut the contents into cubes and remove to a bowl, mix with other fruits and then place back in the pineapple skin
- Do the same with melon, choosing different types of melon so you get a range of colors
- Make a citrus fruit salad with different oranges and grapefruit
- Get red, black and white berries and put into tall serving glasses with a long handled spoon to scoop them out
- Slice apples and pears and put on a small tea plate (squeeze lemon juice over to stop browning)
- Decorate your fruit salads with fresh mint leaves
- Make a "coulis" to drizzle over the fruit or just to decorate the plate – puree berries for a lovely red coulis, melon for a pale coulis to add to dark berries or peaches, mango or nectarines for a lovely orange coulis
- Add some sprinkled nuts and seeds, toast (dry fry in a pan) for a different flavor
- Choose a cream from the recipe list to top a fruit dish and add in more nutrients

Winter Fruit Salad

This is lovely, especially if warmed but very high in sugar, even though it is natural fructose, dried fruits can almost triple in the amount of sugar and calories, so don't have too much! maybe just a large tablespoon on top of porridge or a small bowl to kick start the day with something more substantial to follow such as tofu scramble. Diabetics or those with sugar handling problems beware.

Choose from:

- Figs
- Raisins
- Currants
- Sultanas/raisins
- Prunes
- Apricots
- Dates

Soak these in filtered water overnight, remove from the water in the morning and place in a colander to drain, chop the ones that need chopping, toss with juice of a lime and a fresh chopped apple - top with a little nut cream or just a little soy yogurt and some seeds.

If you want it warm, put in a pan and heat gently for a few minutes.

Smoothies and Juices

Great for breakfast or anytime you need an energy boost

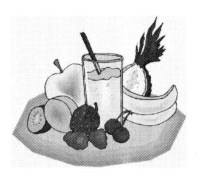

Here are a few recipes, but you know me by now if you have read any of my books, I like people to use their imagination and experiment so mix anything you want - I recommend wheat grass juice but if you have never had it before try it as a shot - see further on in this section.

Mango Smoothie

Per person

Peel and take out the stone of one mango, press fresh oranges or apples to make a cup of juice, blend this together to make a lovely wake up drink.

Melon Smoothie

Per person

Half a melon, peeled, deseed and chopped, fresh orange or apple juice as before, blend up and serve, really hydrating and tasty.

Trisha Stewart

Banana, mango, papaya smoothie

Per person

1 banana, skin removed, 1 mango peeled and de-stoned,1 papaya peeled and de-seeded, 1 cup of fresh pressed apple, orange or grapefruit juice, blend it altogether for a large glass of fabulous nutrition.

Chocolate (carob), Banana and Almond Smoothie

Per person

½ cup raw almonds soaked overnight, remove from liquid and blend with 1 large banana and 1 tbsp of carob powder or cacao nibs, 1 cup of filtered water or juice as above – go on whizz it all up – lush and nutritious.

Berry Smoothie

Per person

2 cups of berries and 1 cup of fresh pressed apple juice – whizz up and drink straight away.

Tips

- To any of the smoothies, add oats, millet, quinoa flakes, ground nuts or seeds for a substantial breakfast; makes it very thick but will satisfy you for a few hours. Use ¼ cup or less per person, depending on which grain you use.

- An avocado adds great nutrition and thickening to any of the above and as it does not have a distinct flavor it will blend in with anything.
- Instead of apple or other juice try some rice milk, nut milks or soy milk or cream but watch those calories mount up.

Juices

Same applies, put whatever you want together but the key here is to have a good juicer as you can lose so many good nutrients in the pulp and through heat produced by a fast machine; as this breaks down the enzymes.

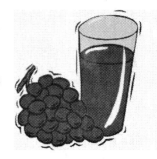

The juices will be great and certainly better for you than bacon and eggs!

All recipes are for one large glassful

	Energizer
2	Apples (preferably those which will give lots of juice, royal gala, pink lady, golden delicious or your preference)
¼	Pineapple
½	Lime or lemon or a piece of each
¼"	Piece of ginger (optional as it gives quite a whack to the taste)
½	Avocado (put a little lemon juice on the other half to stop it going brown)
1"	Piece of cucumber or courgette/zuchinni

1	Handful of parsley

Preparation

- Put everything but the avocado through the juicer
- Blend the avocado and mix everything together
- If you like it chilled put it on ice

Refresher

2	Apples
½	Small carrot or ¼ large one
½	Small beetroot/beets or ¼ large one
1	Broccoli floret
Handful	Mixed greens including spinach and parsley
Small	Piece of courgette/zuchinni or cucumber
Small	Piece of celery (if liked as it can sometimes override other flavors)
Small	Piece of ginger (to taste)
¼	Lemon
Handful	Sprouts such as alfalfa

- Put all the ingredients through the juicer and enjoy!

Healthy Bunch Cook Book

Between Times

2	Apples
1	Carrot
Bunch	Mixed greens
1 Stick	Celery
½	Lemon
¼	Cucumber

- Put it all through the juicer

Sweet and Delicious

¼	Pineapple
½	Avocado
¼	Lime
½"	Piece of Ginger (optional, it packs a punch)
2	Apples

- Put all, except the avocado through the juicer
- Blend the avocado, mix with the other juice ingredients.

Bold as Braass-ica's

Bunch	Greens (spinach, kale, broccoli, cabbage etc)
Small	Bunch parsley
¼	Beetroot/beets (peeled)
2	Apples
1	Carrot
1 stick	Celery

- Put all through the juicer

Simply Orange

110g/ ½ lb   Lovely young carrots
½"   Piece of ginger
1   Small wedge of lime or lemon
30g/1oz   Pomegranate seeds
1   Apple

- Put everything through the juicer, you could add a small bunch or parsley, tarragon or mint

---

Simply Purple

110g/ ½ lb   Lovely young beetroot/beets
½ "   Piece of ginger
1   Small wedge of lime or lemon
30g/1oz   Pomegranate seeds

- Put everything through the juicer, you could add a small bunch or parsley, sage or thyme

---

Wheatgrass

If you are going to add wheatgrass, my advice is to take it as a "shot" in a 1fl oz shot glass and have a little ginger added or a ¼ orange to suck afterwards. It does overpower other juice ingredients so it may ruin what would have been a tasty juice for you. Experiment and find out what works best for you.

Is it worth the effort? Yes! because wheatgrass helps with the following:

1. Purifies and alkalizes the blood
2. Helps prevent or reverse constipation
3. Stimulates the liver
4. Helps to rid the body of toxins
5. Increases enzyme activity in the digestive system
6. Helps to increase the level of good bacteria in the gut
7. Helps the kidneys to cleanse and detoxify

- Take a couple of handfuls of wheatgrass and put through the juicer, it is fabulous to look at so bright and invigorating.

Basically carrots, apples and greens make great juices. All the juices are packed full of vitamins, minerals, bioflavonoids and enzymes you just can't go wrong with your choice. Grow your own wheatgrass as well as sprouts.

Soups

In this section I will show you not just how to make some delicious hot and cold soups but also give you some tips on ringing the changes. Once you have a pan of soup on the go you can have this at anytime, in between meals if you are hungry, for breakfast or other times of the day.

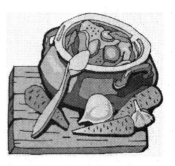

Spiced up Parsnip Potage

Serves 4/6

1 tbsp	Olive Oil or Sunflower Oil
1	Onion (sliced)
675g / 1 ½ lbs	Parsnips (diced)
5ml / 1 ½ tsp	Curry Powder
2ml / ½ tsp	Ground Cumin
900ml /1 ½ pts	Vegetable Stock (freshly made or yeast free/low salt boullion)
150ml / 1/4pt	Soy, rice or coconut milk
Seasoning	Ground black pepper, paprika (optional)
Garnish	Freshly chopped parsley or coriander (cilantro)

Preparation

- Gently fry onion and diced parsnips in the oil for three minutes
- Add curry powder and ground cumin, cook for a further 2 minutes

---

28

- Add stock and bring to a boil, reduce heat and simmer until the vegetables are tender
- Cool soup slightly, blend until smooth
- Return to saucepan, add the soy/rice/coconut milk and reheat to a suitable temperature for eating
- Garnish with parsley or coriander and a sprinkling of paprika (if using)

Tips

- Instead of curry powder and cumin use a recipe from the curry paste section.
- Make sure your parsnips are fresh and young, not "woody" (like wood in the middle)
- Substitute celeriac for the parsnips or a mix of root vegetables.

Carrot and Coriander (Cilantro) Soup

Serves 4/6

1 tbsp	Olive, sunflower or coconut oil
675g / 1 ½ lb	Carrots (chopped)
350g / 12oz	Leeks (chopped) or onions if preferred
1	Large sweet potato
1	Clove of garlic crushed (optional)
1 tbsp	Fresh Lemon juice
Zest	Half lemon
1	Large bunch of coriander (to taste, I love loads!)
900ml /1½ pts	Fresh vegetable stock or yeast free bouillon

Preparation

- Gently sweat off leeks or onions and garlic (if using) for about 1-2 mins until transparent
- Add carrots and sweet potato, cook for a further 2-3 mins
- Add stock and bring to a boil, simmer for 10 minutes or until vegetables are cooked.
- At the end of cooking put the coriander (cilantro) into the pot and leave for a few minutes
- Blend until smooth or if you prefer leave some chunky bits in too
- Return to pan and add lemon juice and lemon zest
- Garnish with fresh chopped coriander (cilantro)
- Season with ground black pepper
- Garnish with fresh chopped coriander (cilantro)

Tips

- This soup can be the base for a range of soups, choose different vegetables to suit. Instead of coriander choose 25gm/1oz of root ginger grated and use orange instead of lemon.

Shroomy Soup

Serves 4

1	tbsp Sunflower, olive or coconut oil
1	Large onion, peeled and finely chopped
350g / 12oz	Mushrooms (button or flat) chopped
570ml / 1pt	Fresh vegetable stock or yeast free bouillon
1 tbsp	Paprika
¼ tsp	Cayenne
3floz / ¼ pt	Soy cream/yogurt

- Ground black pepper to taste and fresh tarragon or parsley

Preparation

- Gently fry onion in oil for a few minutes, add salt to bring out the juices
- Add mushrooms, paprika and cayenne, cook gently for 7-10 Minutes
- Add stock and bring to a boil, simmer for 5 minutes
- Cool soup slightly and blend until smooth
- Return to pan add ground black pepper and cream
- Sprinkle with some fresh Tarragon or Parsley

Tips

- Mushrooms can be very watery so check the amount when frying them off if there looks a lot reduce the amount of stock
- Use dried mushrooms such as shitake (rehydrate) for a change or have a mix of both

---

Tomato and Basil Zuppa

Serves 4

1tbsp	Sunflower or olive oil
2	Cloves of garlic, crushed
675g / 1 ½ lb	Fresh tomatoes, blanched, peeled and coarsely chopped
2 tbsp	Sun dried tomato paste
2ml / ½ tsp	Maple Syrup or agave nectar
600ml / 1pt	Fresh vegetable stock or yeast free bouillon
2 tbsp	Fresh basil, chopped

Preparation

- Gently sweat onions and garlic in oil for 5 minutes until transparent
- Add tomatoes and tomato paste, cook for 1 minute
- Add stock and agave nectar/maple syrup, bring to the boil and simmer for 15 minutes
- Add fresh basil
- Cool slightly
- Strain soup through a sieve into a large mixing bowl and discard the dry residue
- Return to the pan and reheat gently
- Garnish with more fresh basil
- Ground black pepper to taste
- Fresh whole basil leaves to garnish

Tips

- You could add some fresh chillies to the onion mix.
- You could use two 450ml cans of tomatoes instead of fresh for speed

Spring Soup

This soup is especially nice at Spring time, using the young fresh vegetables of the season

Serves 6

1 tbsp	Sunflower, olive or coconut oil
2	Young leeks, sliced diagonally
2	Cloves of garlic, crushed
675g/1 ½ lb	Fresh Tomatoes, blanched, peeled and coarsely chopped
115g/ ¼ lb	Dried borlotti or kidney beans, soaked overnight in cold water
1	Medium carrot, chopped
1	Stick of celery, diced
2	Medium potatoes, diced or small new whole potatoes cut in half
2	Medium courgette (zucchinis), sliced
175g/6oz	Shredded cabbage
115g/4oz	Peas - fresh
900ml/1 ½ pts	Fresh vegetable stock or yeast free vegetable bouillon
2 tbsp	Freshly chopped Basil
1 tbsp	Freshly chopped Parsley
1 tbsp	Small pasta bows or break up some larger pieces
	Fresh ground black pepper to taste

Preparation

- Drain the beans and place in a large pan of water and bring to a boil, boil vigorously for 10 minutes and then

reduce to a simmer for about 1-1.5 hours, drain when cooked and set aside
- Gently sweat the onion and garlic in the oil until the onion is transparent, and then add the carrots, celery and potatoes.
- Cook all the above for 20 minutes
- Add cabbage, zucchini, tomatoes and cook for a further 5 minutes
- Add vegetable stock and bring to a boil, simmer for 10 minutes - adding cooked beans and cooked pasta 5 minutes before the end of cooking
- Add ground black pepper, parsley and basil
- Fresh herbs to garnish

Tips

- Any spring vegetables will be delicious
- Unlike some of the other soups, this recipe is designed to look like a clear broth with the vegetables floating in it

---

Chunky Vegetable and Lentil Soup (great winter warmer)

Serves 4

1 tbsp	Sunflower, olive or coconut oil
2	Onions cut in quarters or eights
2	Cloves of garlic roughly chopped
1	Small pumpkin cubed
2	Large carrots sliced
2	Medium potatoes cubed
115g/4oz	Red, green or brown lentils, washed
900ml/1 ½ pts	Fresh vegetable stock or yeast free bouillon

Ground black pepper to taste
Parsley to garnish

Preparation

- Gently sweat the onion and garlic in oil for 5 minutes until transparent
- Add pumpkin, carrots, potato and cook for five minutes
- Add red lentils and vegetable stock, bring to boil and simmer until vegetables and lentils tender around 25 minutes
- Add black pepper and garnish with parsley

Tips

- Use any lentils, brown, green, puy
- Instead of pumpkin use butternut squash
- Use sweet or white potatoes
- Add any herbs or spices you like for a change

Fruit, Vegetable and Nut Soup

Serves 4-6

1 tbsp	Oil
2	Medium onions, sliced
2	Cloves garlic, crushed
450g/1lb	Carrots, chopped
1	Small potato, chopped
1	Large cooking apple, chopped
900ml/ 1 ½ pts	Fresh vegetable stock or yeast free bouillon
50g/2oz	Broken cashew nuts

Preparation

- Gently sweat onion and garlic in oil, cook for five minutes
- Add carrots, potato, apple and nuts, cook for five minutes
- Add the stock and bring to a boil, reduce heat and simmer until fruit and vegetables are
- tender
- Cool slightly and blend until smooth
- Return to pan, season with black pepper garnish with parsley
- Ground fresh black pepper to taste
- Garnish with parsley

Tips

- Do not blend if you would rather have "bits" in it
- Blending does immerse the flavors

Vichyssoise

Serves 4-6

2 tbsp	Sunflower, olive or coconut oil
450g/1lb	Leeks only white part (reserve the rest for a vegetable stock), sliced diagonally
3	Large banana shallots (6-10 smaller ones) diced
250g/9oz	Potatoes, floury ones such as Maris Piper, peeled and cubed
900ml/ 1 ½ pts	Fresh vegetable stock or yeast free bouillon
300ml/ 1¼ cups	Soy cream

| Pinch | Sea salt and fresh ground black pepper |
| 2 tbsp | Fresh parsley or chives for garnish |

Preparation

- Heat the oil in a pan, add the leeks and shallots and sauté for around 15 minutes until soft but not burnt – put the lid on and turn down low
- Add the potato and cook for a further 2-3 minutes
- Put in the stock, salt and ground black pepper and bring to a boil
- Turn down and simmer for about 15 minutes until the potatoes are cooked through and soft
- Remove from the heat and allow to cool for a few minutes
- Put the soup into a blender with the cream and whizz
- Leave to chill for about four hours or overnight
- Garnish with fresh herbs

Tips

You could use coconut cream instead of soy cream or a nut cream from the recipe section

Trisha Stewart

Roasted Garlic and Squash Soup with Salsa Topping

Serves 4-6

1	Large butternut squash (pumpkin or other squash will do) cut in half and de-seed
2	Full heads (bulbs) of garlic with outer papery skin removed (do not break into cloves)
3	Sprigs of fresh thyme
2	Onions, sliced
5ml/1tsp	Ground coriander
1lt/32floz	Fresh vegetable stock or yeast free bouillon
30-45ml/2-3tbsp	Fresh oregano, chopped
Pinch	Sea salt and fresh ground black pepper

For the Salsa

4	Large ripe tomatoes, full flavor, halved and de-seeded
1	Red pepper, halved and de-seeded
1	Large fresh chilli, halved and de-seeded
2 tbsp	Olive oil
15ml/1 tbsp	Balsamic vinegar

Preparation

- Preheat oven to 220c/425f/gas7
- Put the garlic bulbs on a small sheet of foil
- Put 1 tbsp of the oil over the bulbs and add the thyme, then wrap the foil around them
- Put the two halves of squash, pepper, chilli and tomatoes on a lightly oiled baking tray, lightly rub the

38

vegetables with a little oil, add the foil wrapped garlic to the tray

- Roast in the oven for around 20 minutes
- Take out the tomatoes, chilli and red pepper, set aside
- Reduce the oven heat to190c/375f/gas 5 and leave the squash to cook for another 20-25 minutes until soft, set aside
- Meanwhile, heat the remaining oil in a pan and add the onions and ground coriander, sauté for around 10 minutes until soft
- Take the garlic bulbs and press the soft centre into the onion mix
- Scoop the squash from its outer skin and add to the onion mix
- Add the stock and seasoning and bring to boil, turn down and simmer for around 10 minutes
- Stir in the oregano and allow to cool a little
- Put the soup in a blender and whizz
- Meanwhile skin the pepper and chilli and add to a food processor with the tomatoes and 2 tbsp of olive oil – stir in the balsamic vinegar and seasoning, add a little more oil if needs be
- Warm the soup through when ready to serve and add a dollop of salsa to each bowl, sprinkle on the fresh herbs

Tips

This is a lush and strong tasting soup, will not disappoint those who love taste - the extra work of making a soup like this is worth it

Gazpacho

Serves 4-6

6	Medium ripe tomatoes cut into eights
½	Small/medium cucumber or 1 small courgette/zuchinni diced
1	Green pepper roughly chopped
1	Small red or white onion, diced
2	Cloves of garlic, peeled and minced or diced
200ml/8fl oz	Filtered water
1 tsp	Paprika
1 tsp	Sea salt
½ tsp	Ground cumin
½ tsp	Ground black peppercorns
2 tbsp	Olive oil
2 tbsp	Apple cider vinegar
2 tbsp	Coriander leaves freshly chopped

Preparation

- Place the first 6 ingredients into a blender and whizz
- Add the rest of the ingredients and whizz again
- Put into a suitable container and chill in the refrigerator

Tips

As always anything goes, you can add fresh chillies for a fiery soup, red peppers instead of green and some celery too.

Raw Fiery Soup

Serves 4

450g/1lb	Carrots, topped and tailed and scrubbed
1	Red pepper, roughly chopped
2	Cloves of garlic peeled
1"	Piece of ginger roughly chopped
1	Small red chilli, de-seeded and roughly chopped
1	Avocado, peeled and de-stoned
1 tbsp	Each of fresh mint and basil leaves
1 tbsp	Olive oil
2 tbsp	Tamari sauce
2 tbsp	Apple cider vinegar
½ tsp	Sea salt
	Fresh herbs chopped for garnish

Preparation

- Put all the ingredients into a blender and whizz up
- Chill in the refrigerator

Tips

- Add to each serving some chopped spring onions, cubed avocado, diced peppers, you then have a chunky soup
- For more servings double the quantity and if there is any leftover put into a cooked soup as a base for the vegetable stock or into a chilli, curry, shepherd's pie or anywhere you like, even in a juice, nothing gets wasted in my kitchen.

Lunch boxes

Ok – so there is no bread in here – why – because if you don't know how to make a sandwich then you are really in trouble!

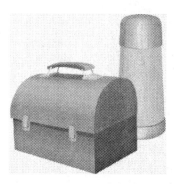

I am going to demonstrate that you can have something different for your lunch box each day of the working week, the only problem you may have is making up all the different recipes on a daily basis so if I were you I would decide on some of the things you really like and get the shopping in for that and then once a week go for something you have either not tried or is a little more challenging to make.

And, you can always remember to use up leftovers from the night before, so if you have cooked rice or nutty rice pilaf, vegetarian paella and so on, those are great cold items to combine into a lunch box, you will soon have your own recipes on the go.

I am drawing on some of the recipes already in the book so will refer you to them by an asterisk*

Lunch Box 1

8floz/1cup	Gazpacho *
225g/1 cup	Tabouleh * per person - so a cupful perhaps
1	Large full salad *per person
1	Small sliced avocado (or half a large one) per person
4 tbsp	French style dressing *
	Large leafy green salad*

Preparation

- Put the salad ingredients into a lunch box with the Tabouleh and dressing in separate containers
- Slice the avocado or cube it when ready to eat
- Pile it onto a plate or eat out of the container

Lunch box snacks

- Fresh fruit
- *Fruit and nut chews

Lunch Box 2

8floz/1cup	Raw and Fiery Soup*
1cup	Bean salad *
1cup	Nutty rice pilaf or plain wholegrain rice
2	Spring onions chopped
	Hand full of chopped chives or basil
	Little sun dried tomato dressing*
	Sprinkling of sunflower seeds
	Handful of mixed leaves

Preparation

- Put each ingredient in a separate container and put together when you are ready to eat

Lunch box snacks
- Fresh Fruit
- Energy Balls*

Lunch Box 3

8floz/1cup	Fruit salad
2-3	Lentil Patties*
8oz/1cup	Slaw *
	Handful of bean sprouts (see sprouting)
1	Large sliced tomato
	Handful of spinach

Preparation

- Layer up starting with spinach, sliced tomatoes, then bean sprouts, slaw and lastly, patties

Lunch box snacks

- Vegetable crudités and hummus*
- Almond and Fig Soft Baked Cookies*

Lunch Box 4

8floz/1cup	Chilled soup of choice
1	Large roasted sweet potato cubed
	Dollop of creamy dressing*
	Huge salad*

Preparation

- Put together when ready to eat

Lunch box snacks
- Fresh fruit
- Vegetable crudités and hummus*

Lunch Box 5

115g/4oz	Marinated tofu*
	Bed of grated beetroot/beets and carrot
	Handful bean sprouts
4tbsp	Dressing from recipe section
	Handful of fresh young spinach leaves

Preparation
- Put into separate containers and throw it together when ready to eat

Lunch box snacks
- Fresh fruit
- Nuts and seeds

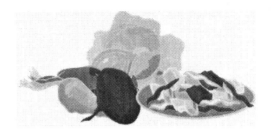

Energizing Lunch Box Treats

These are very high in natural sugar so diabetics, those with sugar handling problems or overweight please leave this section alone and go for the other lovely recipes in the book.

These snacks are really designed to get the children away from those awful snack bars, colored sweets and other commercially made products.

You need very little of these to make an impact on your taste buds and your blood sugar levels.

Energy Balls

Serves 4-6

175g/6oz	Dates
250ml/8fl oz	Filtered water for soaking
50g/2oz	Pecan nuts
2tsp	Tahini
2tsp	Peanut butter

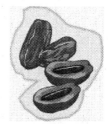

Preparation

- Soak the dates over night, drain and place in a food processor with the other ingredients
- Roughly process and take a tbsp form into a ball
- Use up all the ingredients and place in the refrigerator to chill

---

Tips

- These may not form together too well if your dates are not fully hydrated, if there is a problem it may be a good idea to cook the dates for ten minutes to let the water absorb and then add the other ingredients.
- Try macadamia, brazil or other nuts
- Try apricots instead of dates although they will really need to be hydrated well

---

Carob and Nut Balls

175g/6oz	Ground almonds
75ml/3fl oz	Maple Syrup, date syrup or honey (if not totally vegan)
1 tbsp	Pure almond essence
1 tbsp	Carob powder

Preparation

- Combine the first three ingredients
- Pull together and then take a tablespoon or so and form into a ball, repeat until all the mixture is used up
- Roll the balls into the carob powder and chill in the refrigerator

Tips

- Try melting cacao nibs and rolling the balls in the liquid and then rolling again in some flaked almonds

---

Almond and Fig Soft Baked Cookies

450g/16oz/2cups   Whole almonds soaked overnight
225g/8oz/1cup   Walnuts soaked overnight
750g/24oz/3cups   Dried figs soaked overnight

Preparation

- Preheat the oven to a low temperature of around 120c/250f
- Drain all the ingredients and put into a food processor, coarsely process until the ingredients come together
- Take two tablespoons of the mixture and form into a cookie and place on a baking sheet. Continue to do this until all the mixture has been used.
- Bake in the oven for 1-2 hours. The idea is not to harden these biscuits but just bake enough so they are still soft and luscious to eat.
- Cool and put into an airtight container and keep in the refrigerator for up to one week.

Tips

- Try any nuts and perhaps dates.
- Use these to dip into your homemade ice cream.

This is one of my "bug bears" in the clinic, people wanting something sweet. I never let any of my clients have these high sugar snacks as they usually have some kind of gut dysbiosis, sugar handling problems, diabetes, candida and so on - but in this book I am trying to get the whole family to use whole foods, naturally grown, naturally ripened and eaten as fresh as possible so have conceded to put some in, not really liking it though! BEWARE - high calories.

Other snacks

These can be easy on the waistline and blood sugar levels and much more preferable to the above

- Vegetable Crudités (matchstick vegetables) and a small tub of hummus
- Small soy yogurt and some fresh fruit
- Two pieces of fresh fruit
- 4 Brazil nuts or 6 cashew nuts - not the whole bag!
- Two tablespoons of the granola
- Small handful of seeds
- Homemade potato crisps (very thinly sliced potatoes baked off in the oven till crisp)
- Homemade vegetable crisps (as above) this is where the mandolin comes in nicely!

Salads

I am not going to waste your time by expecting you to look at too many salads; anyone can throw a salad together especially with the amount of leaves and other produce available at the farmers markets and supermarkets today.

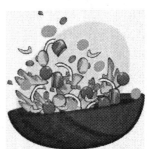

- I would like to warn you right here - if you are buying ready washed salad leaves from the supermarket, PLEASE wash them again, thoroughly; they are washed in chlorinated water!

- Choose as much organic produce as possible to reduce the amount of pesticides you are taking in your food and also buy what is in season and locally to save "air miles".

- Buy from your local farmers market and support the local people. Set up a "grow and swap" system in your neighborhood, you all grow something different and swap so everyone gets a great choice, you don't end up with a whole harvest of tomatoes you can't use up.

- When making dressings PLEASE use good quality and organic, olive oil, balsamic vinegar - cider apple vinegar - soy, tamari sauces. Try them all, you will never want to buy a commercial dressing again

- Start sprouting (see sprouting section); that way you have great protein and lots of enzymes, vitamins and minerals to add to your salads.

- Grow your own herbs in a window box or in pots outside; you will need them in abundance.
- Eat as much raw food as you can every day

Tabouleh *(a great old favorite and very versatile)*

Serves 2-4 Depending on whether you have this for a starter or as a main event

225g/8oz/1 cup	Bulgur wheat
12fl oz/1 ½ cups	Boiling water
3 tbsp	Lemon juice
1 clove	Garlic grated or crushed in a pestle and mortar
Bunch	Fresh mint chopped or ½ tsp dried
¾ tbsp	Olive oil
4/6	Spring onions chopped (use the green if nice)
3	Tomatoes diced
1	Small cucumber diced
4oz/½ cup	Olives if liked, pitted are best
Bunch	Parsley some chopped some left for garnish

Preparations

- Combine the bulgur wheat and water, stir and let sit for 30 minutes to re-hydrate
- Stir after the 30 minutes to check there is no moisture, if there is drain off
- Add lemon juice, garlic and oil
- Add the remaining ingredients and stir

Tips

- This is nice if left to sit for a while so that the flavors can combine.
- Nice to have in a lunchbox
- Good as a salad combo with lentil and bean salads and grated carrots and beetroot/beets

---

Roasted Root Salad

Serves 6

Depending if you just have this on its own or accompanying another dish

4	Red onions (medium) quartered
8	Raw baby beetroot/beets scrubbed and trimmed
900g/2lb	Potatoes – small or about the size of the beetroot/beets
900g/2lb	Pumpkin (or butternut squash), deseeded and cubed
3tbsp	Olive oil
2 tbsp	Lemon or lime juice
2 tbsp	Fresh oregano chopped roughly
1 tbsp	Fresh thyme chopped finely
½ tsp	Sea salt

Dressing

3tbsp	Olive oil
4 tbsp	Apple cider vinegar
2 tbsp	Coarse grain mustard

Directions

- Preheat the oven to 200c/400f/Gas mark 6
- Lay the vegetables out on a large baking tray
- Put the other ingredients (not the dressing) into a bowl a mix
- Pour over the vegetables, mix with clean hands to coat each piece
- Bake in the oven for about 45 mins- make sure the vegetables are cooked
- Make the dressing by placing all the ingredients in a bowl to whisk or in a small jar with a lid on and shake.
- Let the vegetables cool and then pour on the dressing and add some coarse ground black pepper and garnish with some fresh herbs

Tips

- This can be eaten while still warm; I personally prefer it like that. But, you can leave it to get cold and even store it in the refrigerator for the next day. If you do that, don't dress the vegetables until you are ready to eat or the whole thing will be too soggy.
- Vary the vegetables, but try to get ones that respond well to roasting and ring the changes with fresh herbs too.
- You could serve this with a lovely crisp green raw salad or on a bed of wilted spinach

Avocado, Pear and Strawberry Salad

Serves 2

(Just double up on the
quantities if you have more
people)

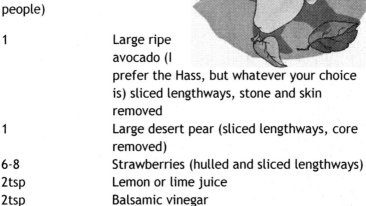

1	Large ripe avocado (I prefer the Hass, but whatever your choice is) sliced lengthways, stone and skin removed
1	Large desert pear (sliced lengthways, core removed)
6-8	Strawberries (hulled and sliced lengthways)
2tsp	Lemon or lime juice
2tsp	Balsamic vinegar

Preparation

- Using individual tea plates, lay half the avocado slices on the bottom, the pear next and tumble the strawberries over the top
- Mix the lemon/lime juice and balsamic vinegar and dress the salad

Tips

- This will make a lovely starter or even a pudding
- Place the ingredients on a bed of spinach or rocket
- Blend/crush all the ingredients and chill into a mousse
- Just have the avocado and add sweet cherry tomatoes and serve on a bed of spinach or rocket

The Best Slaw you will ever taste!

(You will never buy a commercial mayo
loaded one again)

Serves 4-6

225g/8oz/1cup	Red cabbage, shredded finely
1	Medium cucumber, diced or cut into shreds
1	Large, grated carrot
1	Small grated onion or shred some spring onions
1 tsp	Each cumin seeds and ground cumin
1	Large lemon or lime (or both) juiced
2	Large tomatoes diced
2	Cloves of garlic crushed in a pestle and mortar with a little sea salt
2fl oz/ ¼ cup	Olive oil

Preparation

- Put first four ingredients into a large bowl
- Mix the olive oil, cumin seeds, ground cumin, lemon/lime juice, minced garlic/sea salt
- Pour the dressing over and mix with clean hands to coat the vegetables

Tips

- Great stuffed into jacket potatoes
- Good as a salad combo with bean salad and rice salad
- Use white cabbage to ring the changes

- Try grated celeriac instead of carrots or a bit of both
- If you do fancy a mayo type slaw, go to the dressings section of the book and then omit the olive oil and lemon juice from this recipe

---

The Best Leafy Salad ever

(If you can't find all the ingredients you may have to improvise!)

Serves 4 - 6 depending on how you are serving it

Where I have indicated a handful, it depends on the size of your hands, me, I would cup both hands together and fill them, a man with large hands may find one handful enough

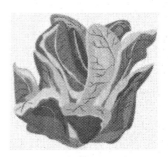

Ingredients

- Large handful each of red lettuce (Lollo rosso or similar), spinach, rocket, Chinese leaves.
- A small bunch each of basil, parsley, oregano, thyme, sage and coriander (de-stem and roughly tear)
- Toss it all together in a large bowl with clean hands

Tips

- I know that looks simple and it is, but the taste and the aromas will delight you, all you need is a dressing of your choice, so go look in the dressings section of the book

- Serve with anything that requires a salad or just have between meals to get some great enzymes in.
- You could even juice it all!

Raw Vegetable Salad

(Great for between meals or as a side dish or starter)

Serves 4 Depending on how you are using it.

2	Carrots cut into very thin sticks (julienne) using a sharp knife or a mandolin
1	Courgette/zucchini, cut as above
225g/8oz/1cup	Bean sprouts, mung are nice or any others that you have sprouted or bought
225g/8oz/1cup	Fresh green beans, runner or French or similar, sliced very thinly
225g/8oz/1cup	Shredded broccoli

Preparations

- Put all the vegetables into a large bowl and toss with clean hands
- Top with a dollop of hummus, guacamole or dressing of choice

Tips

- Munching through that lot will keep you occupied for a while and exercise your jaws, deliver some top class enzymes, vitamins and minerals too.

Beetroot/beets Salad

Serves 4 as a side salad

2	Large grated Beetroot/beets
1"	Grated fresh ginger root
1 tsp	Fresh lemon juice
1 tbsp	Tamari sauce
1 tsp	Honey (If not totally Vegan) or maple syrup

- Throw it all in a large bowl and mix with clean hands

Tips

This is a good combo mix for other salads.

- Great color to add to any dish
- Slice some oranges to garnish
- Throw a few pine nuts or seeds over the top
- Ring the changes with other root vegetables

Bean Salad with a roasted red pepper and chilli dressing

Serves 4 (ish)

350g/12oz/1.5 cups	Beans - Flageolet, haricot or a mix of any beans soaked overnight in cold water
1	Large red pepper
4 tbsp	Olive oil
1	Large clove garlic crushed

Bunch	Fresh coriander (or other herb) leaves (small bunch will do the job)
1 tbsp	Balsamic vinegar
2	Fresh red chilis, de-seeded and chopped

Preparation

- Put the beans into a large pan of water and bring to a boil, skim off any froth, turn down and simmer for 1.5 – 2 hours depending on the type of beans
- Heat the oven to 200c/400f/Gas 6
- Put the whole pepper on a lightly oiled baking tray and lightly brush with a little olive oil
- Roast for 30 minutes
- Remove, allow to cool and peel off the skin, cut in half and de-seed, leave aside
- Heat the remaining oil in a pan, cook garlic and chillies for 1 minute
- Add the pepper, herbs and balsamic vinegar
- Put the beans into a bowl and pour over the dressing and mix to combine all the flavors

Tips

- Instead of adding chilli and coriander add sun dried tomatoes and basil
- Whenever a recipe calls for beans you can cook up a load, put into small containers and freeze, this way you will always have some handy
- You can use canned beans but do get the salt and sugar free ones and rinse well

Japanese Style Salad

This is stunning to look at - the black strands of Hijiki combined with the red of the radishes and green of the cucumber or zucchini, as well as being full of nutrients

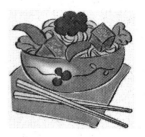

Serves 2-4

15g/ ½ oz	Hijiki (dried)
250g/9oz/1 ¼ cups	Radishes, sliced
1	Small cucumber or zucchini/courgette (julienned/cut into thin strips)
75g/3oz/ ½ cup	Bean sprouts

Dressing	
15ml/1 tbsp	Each of sunflower and toasted sesame oil
2tsps	Lemon or lime juice
5ml/1 tsp	Tamari sauce
30ml/1 tbsp	Apple cider vinegar
1 tsp	Chopped fresh red chilli
15ml/1 tbsp	Mirin (or rice wine or add another tbs of apple cider vinegar)
6	Shredded spring onions to garnish

Preparation

- Soak the hijiki in a bowl of cold water for 15 minutes, drain and repeat three/four times, the yield should be around three times the dried amount, be totally hydrated and soft
- Put the dressing ingredients into a blender or screw top jar and shake or whiz; Set aside

- Put the bean sprouts, radishes, cucumber (or courgette/zucchini) into a bowl
- Put hijiki and dressing ingredients into the bowl of vegetables and mix well with clean hands or a couple of forks

Tips

- This looks dramatic and tastes delicious but if you are not sure about or have never tasted sea vegetables – make a small amount, it's easy to make and you can make more next time.
- This makes a great starter, or as part of a salad combo.

Louisiana Salad

Serves 4-6

225g/8oz	Just ripe, de-stoned and peeled avocados
1 tbsp	Lemon juice
225g/8oz	Fresh pineapple
125g/4oz	Each small diced red pepper and celery
225g/8oz	Cooked wholegrain rice

Dressing

1 tbsp	Apple cider vinegar
6tbsp	Olive oil
1 tbsp	Lemon juice
1 tsp	Red chilli, finely chopped
1	Garlic clove, crushed

| 1tbs | Creole spices* (less if you don't like this too spicy)(see recipe) |

Preparation

- Make sure you have the rice cooked
- Chop the avocado, place in a bowl and put some of the lemon juice on it to stop it going brown
- Put the peppers and celery into a bowl and add the drained avocado to the mixture
- Add the cooked rice but don't mix in until you have the dressing ready
- Mix the dressing ingredients in a screw top jar or a blender
- Gently mix everything together so as not to smash the avocado
- Serve on a bed of leaves

Hawaiian Rice Salad

Serves 4-6

225g/8oz	Wholegrain basmati rice, cooked and chilled
½	Medium cucumber, diced
3	Firm tomatoes, diced
½	Small red pepper, diced
½	Small green pepper, diced
115g/4oz	Green peas
115g/4oz	Corn niblets
115g/4oz	Sultanas/raisins soaked in 1 cup or orange juice for 1 hour, or 3 slices of pineapple, diced
4fl oz/ ½ cup	Cup of Italian dressing* (see recipe section)

| 2 | Cloves garlic, crushed |
| 4 tbsp | Chopped parsley |

Preparation

- Heat a little oil in a pan and sauté off the garlic, set aside
- Place all the ingredients (except dressing) in a large bowl
- Toss the salad with the dressing and serve on the lettuce leaves
- Crisp lettuce leaves for decoration

Spanish Style Rice Salad

Serves 4-6

250g/8oz/1cup	Wholegrain basmati or wild rice
1 bunch	Spring onions, sliced thinly
1	Each of red and yellow (or green) pepper, de-seeded and sliced
3	Tomatoes, chopped
2 tbsp	Chopped fresh coriander
8-12	Olives (small or 6 larger ones halved)

Dressing

3tbsp	Olive oil
1 tsp	Grainy mustard
1 tbsp	Lemon or lime juice
1	Clove of garlic crushed

| 1 tbsp | Fresh tarragon or other fresh herb, chopped finely |

Preparation

- Cook the rice in a pan of water for around 20 minutes until soft to touch, drain and rinse in cold water - set aside and leave to cool
- Put the other ingredients (except dressing) into a bowl and add the cold rice
- Put the dressing ingredients in a blender and whizz till nicely blended
- Pour the dressing over the rice and vegetables and mix in well

Tips

- Replace the rice with rice pasta
- Replace the dressing with an oriental one from the dressing section of the book

Dressings and more...

Sauces – Mayo– Cream – Cheeze – Nut Butter - Salsa – Spreads

This section is dedicated to providing you with a range of dips, dressings, sauces, cream and cheeze. I have a "tip" below each recipe to help you utilize the recipe to its maximum. There are no hard and fast rules in cooking or non cooking, it's all about you and your taste and texture

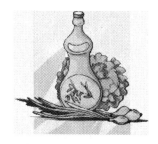

preferences, so if you don't have the exact ingredients, don't worry, be adventurous, don't hold back, get creating dishes that will not only fill you full of nutrients but wake up your taste buds and energize your body and mind.

Tzatsiki

Serves 4-6

350ml/12fl oz	Soy yogurt
1	Medium cucumber, diced or grated
20ml/1 tbsp	Fresh lemon or lime juice
10ml/2 tsp	Olive oil
3-5	Cloves garlic, crushed
2 tbsp	Fresh chopped mint or parsley
	Ground fresh black pepper to taste

Preparation

- Line a sieve with cheese cloth, place over a bowl and pour yogurt into it and drain for 2 hours
- Empty the drained yogurt into a bowl and add the cucumber, garlic, lemon/lime juice and pepper and half the mint/parsley, combine well
- Garnish with the rest of the mint/parsley and serve

Tips

This is a very versatile Greek meze dish; it can be a sauce, dip or dressing.

Hummus

Serves 6

225g/8oz	Chickpeas, soaked overnight in plenty of cold water
2-4 tbsp	Water from the cooked chickpeas
3 or more	Cloves of garlic, crushed
2	Lemons, juiced (or a mix of lemon, lime, orange)
½ tsp	Ground cumin
3 tbsp	Tahini

- To garnish, olive oil, ¼ tsp paprika, 1 tsp fresh parsley, black olives

Preparation

- Drain the soaked chick peas and place them in a large pan of water, bring to a boil and then simmer until they are soft, 1-1.5hrs. Remove any foam that forms during cooking

- Drain the chickpeas and reserve 2-4 tbsp cooking liquid
- Place the chickpeas, oil, lemon juice, garlic and tahini into a blender and blend until smooth, adding a little of the cooking liquid to get the right consistency
- Add more lemon juice to taste
- Pour hummus into a serving dish and garnish

Tips

- This dish is a Middle Eastern dip or spread
- Add roasted vegetables to the blend
- Blend some sun dried tomatoes (refreshed) and stir in
- Add some chopped fresh herbs
- Can be a dressing or a dip

Guacamole

Serves 4-6

Ingredients

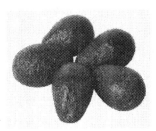

4	Ripe, medium avocados, peeled and stoned
10ml/2tsp	Fresh lemon or lime juice
1-2	Cloves of garlic, crushed
	Fresh ground black pepper and chilli powder to taste/optional
	Parsley to garnish

Preparation

- Put all the ingredients, except seasoning and garnish into a blender, puree, season to taste and chill in a refrigerator for a couple of hours
- Pour into a suitable container and garnish

Tips

- This dish is a Mexican dip, spread or dressing
- If you just want to make a small amount use 1 avocado per person and reduce the rest of the ingredients

---

Quick Tahini Dressing

2	Cloves of garlic, crushed
120ml/4fl oz	Tahini
120ml/4fl oz	Water
2	Lemons, juiced

Preparation

- Put everything into a blender and whizz up, add more lemon juice or water for a thinner sauce or less for a thicker one

Tips

- Excellent as a salad dressing or with rice and vegetables

Tarragon and Walnut Dressing

4 tbsp	Safflower oil (sunflower or other oil will be fine too)
2 tbsp	Walnut oil
2 tbsp	Apple cider vinegar
1 tbsp	Orange or lemon juice
3-4 tbsp	Fresh chopped tarragon

Preparation

- Place everything in a blender and whizz, you have a perfect dressing

Tips

- Great on avocado or dessert pears

Hot and Green Dressing

1	Large or two small avocados (I prefer the little black Hass), peeled and de-stoned
2	Medium ripe tomatoes cut into quarters
1 tbsp	Olive oil
1 tbsp	Lemon Juice
1	Fresh red chilli de-seeded and roughly chopped
1	Small red onion, roughly chopped
1	Clove garlic, peeled and roughly chopped

Preparation

- Put all the ingredients into a blender and whiz

Tips

- Omit the fresh red chili and add a ¼ tsp ground chili powder

---

Vegan Mayo – *nothing like you have had before!*

2fl oz/ ¼ cup	Lemon Juice
2	Cloves garlic, crushed
3	Stalks of celery, roughly chopped
3	Fresh chopped tomatoes
1	Chopped red or green pepper
1	Small chopped onion
2 tbsp	Minced or finely chopped fresh parsley and thyme
300g/10oz	Cashew nuts (preferably soaked in water overnight)

Preparation

- Put all the ingredients in a blender and whizz until creamy, you may need to add a little filtered water to make to the consistency you like

Tips

- This will keep in the fridge for up to 3 days
- Ring the changes with the herbs and try basil and oregano or another combo

- Use other vegetables that will blend well
- Spice it up and put in some minced red chillies
- Great with potato wedges, as a topping for a jacket potato, as well as salad and for dipping crudités!

Nut Butter

| 200g/7 oz | Any nuts or peanuts or mix of nuts (preferably soaked in water overnight) |
| 2fl oz/ ¼ cup | Liquid – this could be freshly squeezed orange juice, apple juice, coconut water or even just filtered water |

Preparation

- Grind the nuts in a coffee grinder or similar
- Place nuts in a blender carefully pour in the liquid a little at a time so as not to get the mixture to sloppy, it needs to be "scraped out" and spreadable

Tips

- This will keep in the fridge for a few days
- For a spicy butter to add to any dish, mince some chillies, garlic and blend
- You could use your Creole spice mix* to blend in too
- This is a great alternative to using dairy butter
- If you make it a little runny you could use it as a nut sauce

Cream

200g/7 oz	Nuts, again your choice but I like cashews (soaked overnight)
4fl oz/½ cup	Fresh squeezed orange juice
4fl oz/½ cup	Filtered water
1 tbsp	Maple syrup or honey (not vegan)
A few drops	Either almond extract or vanilla essence

Preparation

- Drain the nuts and place in a blender with the rest of the ingredients, making sure everything mixes well
- Check the consistency and taste, try to think about what you will be having this with and adjust for sweetness
- Check the amount of water you are adding and add slowly to get the consistency you like

Tips

- You could use this on top of porridge or muesli
- Put into a piping bag and swirl over a fruit salad
- For a savory or sour cream omit the maple syrup and add tamari sauce, garlic and spices or black pepper, mashed avocado makes it a lovely color! A great topping for a salad or some steamed vegetables.

Cheeze - I know it's not dairy!

200g/7oz	Pumpkin or other seeds such as sesame and sunflower, a mix is nice (soaked overnight in filtered water)
1 tbsp	Each minced ginger, garlic and red or green pepper
1 bunch	Fresh parsley roughly chopped
2fl oz/4 tbsp	Tamari sauce
1-2 tbsp	Olive oil
4fl oz/ ½ cup	Fresh squeezed lemon juice

Preparation

- Drain seeds and blend with the rest of the ingredients

Tips

- Will keep for a couple of days in the fridge
- Vary the types of seeds to create a different flavor
- Add in some spices and chilies to have hot cheeze
- Use orange juice for a change
- Add different herbs such as coriander, thyme and rosemary or basil and oregano
- Go plain and take out the peppers and tamari sauce

Red Pepper Sauce

200g/7oz/ ¾ cup	Tinned tomatoes or passata
½	Green pepper, diced
4 tbsp	Onion, diced
½	Fresh red chilli, de-seeded and diced
1 tbsp	Fresh coriander, chopped
½ tsp	Each ground coriander and cumin

Preparation

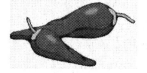

- Put everything in the blender and whizz till smooth
- Heat through gently for around 15-20 minutes

Tips

- If you want this sauce hotter, add more chillies

Peanut Sauce (Satay)

115g/4oz	Natural, unsalted peanuts
1 ½ tbsp	Coconut oil or groundnut oil
3	Medium shallots or small onions, diced
2	Cloves garlic, crushed
1"	Fresh root ginger, grated
2 tbsp	Apple cider vinegar
2 tbsp	Tamari
1 tbsp	Maple syrup
1-2	Fresh red chillies, de-seeded and diced
3 tbsp	Filtered water

Preparation

- Heat the oil in a frying pan and sauté off the shallots or onions, garlic and ginger for 5 minutes
- Add the peanuts and stir into the mix and sauté off for around 2 minutes
- Place the mix and rest of the ingredients, except the water, into a blender or food processor and whizz gently adding a little water to get a sauce consistency
- Place into a pan or jug for use later

Tips

- Make this as hot as you like with the addition of more chillies

---

Sweet and Sour Sauce

About **8 portions** depending on how you use it

225ml/8fl oz/1cup	Fresh pressed orange juice
110ml/4fl oz/½ cup	Tamari sauce
1.5" piece	Fresh root ginger, grated
3-4	Cloves of garlic, crushed
2 tbsp	Maple syrup or honey (not for vegan)
4tsp	Sesame oil
4 tbsp	Corn flour/corn starch

Preparation

- Dissolve the corn flour/corn starch in a little water to become a paste
- Whizz the rest of the ingredients in a blender
- Add the corn flour/corn starch and set aside

Tips

- This sauce will keep in the refrigerator for a few days
- Add to stir fry vegetables
- Add chillies if you want it hotter

Quick Butter Bean, Sweet Red Pepper and Basil Pate

Serves 4

425g/15oz	can butter or lima beans
1 tbsp	freshly squeezed lemon juice
1	Garlic clove, crushed
4	Sprigs basil
1	Small sweet red pepper, deseeded and very finely chopped

Preparation

- Drain and rinse beans under cold water.
- Put in a food processor or blender with lemon juice, garlic and basil and whiz to a purée.
- Mix in sweet pepper
- Place in serving dish

Tips

- This is the basis for any pate so you could use other beans or lentils, other vegetables, add in garlic or ginger and some tamari sauce

---

Italian Salad Dressing

2 tbsp	Fresh lemon juice
6tbsp	Olive oil
1 tsp	Paprika
1	Garlic clove, crushed
1 tsp	Agave nectar or maple syrup (optional)
Pinch	Each: dried oregano, black pepper, dried sage and dill. If fresh herbs are available use twice the amount

Preparation

- Place all the ingredients in a blender for a few seconds, pour dressing into a suitable container and refrigerate

Tips

- Will keep in the fridge for up to a week

Oriental Dressing

6 tbsp	Olive oil
2 tsp	Lemon juice
4 tsp	Soy sauce
½ tsp	Grated root ginger

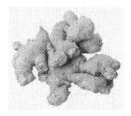

Preparation

- Put all the ingredients in a jar or a blender and shake of whizz

Tips

- Will keep in the fridge for up to a week

French dressing

Ingredients

6 tbsp	Olive oil
2 tsp	Lemon juice
2 tbsp	Cider vinegar

Preparation

- Put all the ingredients in a jar or blender and shake or whiz

Tips

- Variations on the above could include crushed garlic, balsamic vinegar, mustard and any fresh herbs you may like.
- Will keep in the fridge for about a week

Sun dried Tomato Dressing

120ml/4fl oz	Olive oil
1	Lemon juiced
1 tbsp	Apple cider vinegar
2 tbsp	Sun dried tomato puree or sun dried tomatoes (rehydrated)
1 tsp	Each cumin, allspice, oregano, marjoram and a little cayenne pepper

Preparation

- Put all the ingredients into a blender and whizz

Tips

- Will keep in the fridge for about a week
- Use spices for a different taste

Creole Seasoning

2 tbsp	onion powder
2 tbsp	garlic powder
2 tbsp	dried oregano
2 tbsp	dried basil

1 tbsp	dried thyme leaves
1 tbsp	black pepper
1 tbsp	white pepper
1 tbsp	cayenne pepper
1 tbsp	celery seed
5 tbsp	sweet paprika

Mix all of these into an airtight pot and use wherever you need something really well seasoned. This will add a kick to any sauce, gravy, casserole or dressing.

Salsa

Serves 4-6

450g/1lb/2cups	Chopped fresh tomatoes
4-6 tsp	Fresh chopped coriander
1-2	Fresh red chillies, finely chopped
60g/2.5oz/ ½ cup	Minced red onion
3-6	Cloves of garlic crushed or chopped finely

Preparation

- Put all the ingredients in a bowl and mix with either two forks or your hands.

Tips

- If you prefer this hotter add more chillies or less hot, reduce the amount.

- You can blend part of the mix to have more of a sauce than chutney.
- Add in anything you like, maybe some chopped celery or peppers.

Main Courses

I have no idea on who eats what for lunch or dinner or what you call a main course, lunch, snack or whatever. In my clinic experience everyone is different, so what you will see is a variety of dishes which you can eat at any time of the day to suit your activity, i.e. exercising, sitting in a meeting or having friends around for lunch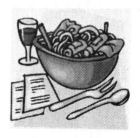
– there is something for every occasion – don't forget the curry and salad section too!

Fast Food Burger

Makes 6-8

1	medium onion, peeled and chopped
1	large peeled garlic clove or to taste
1	medium carrot, peeled and coarsely grated (about 60g prepared weight)
420g/15oz	can 'no-salt no-sugar' red kidney beans, drained and rinsed in a colander under cold running water or a mix of other beans
225g/8oz	Smoked or natural tofu or marinated*
85g/3oz	Sunflower seeds
1	Small bunch parsley
2 tsp	Yeast free vegetable bouillon powder

Preparation

- Preheat the oven to 220C/Gas Mark 7.
- Line a large baking tray with baking parchment

- Place all the ingredients in a food processor and blend roughly-do not puree.
- Grab a handful of mixture and form into a ball and place on the baking tray. Press with fingertips to make a burger shape. How many you will get depends on the size burger you would like.
- Bake for 25 minutes, do not overcook

Tips

- You could fry these in a little oil or put on the barbecue
- These are great hot or cold or served with Vegan Mayo (see recipe), salad and potato wedges

---

French *Cassoulet*

Serves 4-6

(If you are lucky enough to have leftovers, see tips)

1	Large onion, sliced
2	Clove of garlic
1 tbsp	Olive oil
1	Large aubergine/eggplant, cut into cubes (salted, drained, and blotted dry if desired)
2	Red peppers, sliced
6-8	Cherry or plum tomatoes, left whole
2	Courgette/zucchini, sliced
350g/12floz	Passata
	A little sea salt

Trisha Stewart

Herbes de Provence dried which should be a
mix of Rosemary, Basil, Marjoram, Savory,
and Thyme

I also like to put in fresh Basil it has such a wonderful smell and
taste. Add towards the end.

Preparation

- Sauté onion and garlic in olive oil
- Add the aubergine/eggplant and sauté for a
  few minutes.
- Add the peppers, tomatoes and zucchini and
  cook off for a few minutes.
- Add herbs and passata.
- Let cook over medium-low heat for 30 minutes,
  stirring occasionally.

Tips

- Serve hot as a main dish, or cold as a side dish.
- This is a very handy recipe as you can stuff it
  into jacket (sweet or white) potato, or stuff
  any vegetable that is "stuffable."
- Serve with rice or rice pasta
- Serve with vegetables or a huge green salad

Lentil Rissoles

Serves 4-6

115g/4oz/1cup	Lentils, (red/green/brown) cooked in 2 cups water
2	Small to medium carrots grated
1	Medium onion, finely chopped
1	Red or green pepper finely diced
1	Courgette/zucchini finely diced
300g/10oz/1.5cups	Medium/fine oats
60g/2oz	Tomato paste
1 tbsp	Italian seasoning
2-4 tbsp	Olive oil or coconut oil

Preparation

- Bring water to boil and put lentils in. Bring back to simmer for about 15 minutes or until just soft. Drain and set aside
- Heat 1 tbsp oil in a pan and sauté the onions until they look translucent, do not brown
- Add carrots, peppers and courgette/zucchini cook until just softening, add the oats, tomato paste and Italian seasoning, set aside
- Put the lentils and the other ingredients into a bowl and mix.
- Shape them into rolls, rounds, squares or whatever suits you.
- Fry them in a little oil or put them on the barbecue

Tips

You can add spices to these for a change and try different vegetables such as celery or spinach, sweet potato mashed with the lentil mixture, they are great hot or cold.

Giant Bean Stew

Named as such because my sister always thought my stews were so chunky that a giant was coming to dinner!

Serves 4-6

110g/4oz	Each dried chick peas, butter beans, red kidney beans (or any mix), soaked overnight in separate bowls in loads of water
300ml/½ pt	Liquid reserved from the bean cooking water
1 tbsp	Olive oil or coconut oil
225g/ ½ lb	Onions, roughly chopped
2-3	Cloves of garlic, sliced
350g/ ¾ lb	Button mushrooms, halved or quartered
2	Red peppers or a red and green, de-seeded and roughly cut into chunky bits
1	Bulb of fennel, sliced into rounds, then cut across the centre to make crescents
6-8	Cherry tomatoes
400g/1lb	Smoked tofu (or used marinated from recipe section)
2 tbsp	Tamari sauce
100ml/3fl oz/ ½ cup	Sun dried tomato puree
Bunch	Fresh, roughly chopped parsley

1 tbsp	Dried herbs de Provence
1 tbsp	Yeast free vegetable stock
1 tbsp	Grainy mustard

Preparation

- Drain the beans and place in pans of cold water, bringing each to a boil, turn down and simmer for 45 minutes to 1.5 hours depending on the bean, you should be able to squeeze them between finger and thumb without them falling apart but soft enough to eat
- Meanwhile, heat the oil in a large pan and sauté off the onions and garlic until soft, about five minutes, medium heat, do not frazzle them
- Add the peppers, fennel and herbs and cook for a further ten minutes
- Add the mushrooms and tomatoes and cook for a further five minutes
- Add the drained beans and enough water to just about cover the contents of the pan
- Add the vegetable stock, tomato puree and grainy mustards and cook for about twenty minutes on a low heat so everything is bubbling slowly
- Meanwhile, get the sliced marinated or smoked tofu and put under the grill or on a griddle for a minute each side (this stops it from falling apart in the stew)
- Put the slices into the stew and cook for about ten minutes
- Stir in the parsley and leave to stand for ten minutes

Tips

- Soak and cook twice as many beans and reserve the rest for a bean salad
- Choose different herbs for a change of flavor

Quick Bean Casserole

Serves 4-6

2	Large onions sliced
1 tbsp	Olive oil
2	Cloves garlic diced (or to taste)
4	Tomatoes sliced
1	Courgette/zucchini sliced
4 Tbsp	Tahini
500ml/16fl oz	Vegetable stock from yeast free bouillon or homemade stock
	Mixed beans such as Haricot, Kidney, Flageolet, Butter (cooked) if using canned ensure sugar and salt free and rinse thoroughly
2 tsp	Mixed dried herbs such as Italian or Provence
1	Large Sweet Potato sliced
	Fresh herbs to dress

Preparation

- In a large sauté pan, put a little olive oil and sauté the sliced onions till transparent

- Add the garlic, sauté for a minute or two
- Add the tomatoes and courgette/zuchinni
- Add the beans
- Mix the Tahini, herbs and vegetable stock and add to the mixture, do not make it too wet at this stage
- Put into a casserole dish
- Place the sweet potato on top
- Bake in the oven on 170c 325f gas 3 for about an hour

Tips

- You can leave it all in the sauté pan, put the potato on top and simmer with a lid on, baked in the oven is nicer though
- You may need to add a little stock if the casserole gets to look dry
- Try some fresh herbs instead of dried
- Try ginger and spices instead of herbs

Vegetable paella

Serves 4-6

2 tbsp	Olive oil
225g/8oz	Chopped onion
2 cloves	Garlic, crushed
225g/8oz	Courgette (zucchini)- sliced
115g/4oz	Each red pepper, green pepper, mange tout (sugar snap peas)
2	Sticks of celery, chopped

225g/8oz	Wholegrain Basmati rice (you can use traditional Arborio rice)
600ml/1pt	Vegetable stock, fresh or yeast free bouillon
75g/3oz	Roughly chopped almonds or whole pine nuts
Large pinch	Saffron, soaked in a little water
6-8	Olives

Preparation

- Sweat off the onions and garlic in the oil for a few minutes until translucent
- Add the rice and cook over a moderate heat for two minutes, stirring, the rice should look translucent
- Add the stock and the saffron in its water and bring to a boil, reduce heat and simmer for approximately 30 minutes without the lid on
- Add the vegetables, if required, a little more stock, cover and cook for 15 minutes making sure the rice is soft and the vegetables cooked
- Place in a serving dish
- Sprinkle the almonds and olives on to the paella

Tips

- Choose any selection of vegetables
- Serve with a lovely big green salad
- Great cold for the lunchbox

Nut Roast

Serves 4-6

1tbs	Olive oil or coconut oil
450g/16oz	Mixed nuts, finely chopped
350/12 oz	Tomatoes, blanched, peeled & chopped or tinned 1 large onion
1	Clove of garlic diced
115g/4oz	Fresh mushrooms, chopped
1 tsp	Dried basil and dried oregano or other mixed herbs to taste
350g/12oz	Cooked millet or quinoa

Preparation

- Preheat oven to 425 F (220) gas 7
- Lightly oil a loaf tin
- Sauté the onion and garlic in a little olive oil until the onion is transparent
- Place these in a mixing bowl and add the rest of the ingredients
- Turn the mixture into the prepared loaf tin, smoothing the surface with the back of a spoon. Place the tin in oven and bake for 30-40 minutes

Tips

- Serve with an onion gravy made from sliced onions sautéed in olive oil, 350ml of vegetable stock, 1 tbsp tomato paste, 1 tsp mustard, bring to the boil, then turn down and simmer till cooked.
- Vary the nuts or just use one kind, say cashew as they are nice and creamy

- Use a variety of mushrooms

Bean and Lentil Loaf

400g/14oz	Cooked red kidney beans or other lentils
1	Large onion, chopped
2	Cloves of garlic, crushed (less if you prefer)
2	Sticks of celery, chopped
1	Large carrot, grated
115g/4oz	Nuts, any type, coarsely chopped
1 tbsp	Olive oil or coconut oil
2 tbsp	Sun dried tomato puree
1 tsp	Ground cumin
1 tsp	Ground coriander
1 tsp	Chilli powder
350g/12oz	Cooked millet or quinoa

Preparation

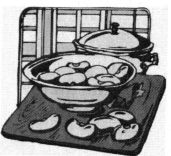

- Pre-heat oven to 180c/350f/gas4
- Heat the oil in a pan and sauté off the onion and garlic for about 5 minutes until soft
- Place the beans in a bowl and mash or whizz in a blender, this depends if you want a smooth loaf or one with texture to it
- Put the beans, lentils, cooked grains, onion and garlic into a bowl
- Add the rest of the ingredients and mix well together
- Put the whole lot into a lightly oiled loaf tin and cook in the oven for about 45minutes to 1 hour

---

Tips

- Vary the beans and vegetables and spices
- Leave to go cold and slice, great for the lunchbox

Parsnip and Carrot Risotto (this is one of my favorites)

Serves 4-6

350g/12oz	Rice (use Arborio if you want to be authentic)
1 tbsp	Olive oil
1 large	Sliced onion
1 clove	Garlic diced
2/3	Carrots (medium size) cut into sticks
2	Parsnips (not the large woody ones) cut into sticks
1 liter	Or more of yeast free vegetable stock Bunch Fresh coriander chopped (or other fresh herbs)

Preparation

- Sauté the onion in a little olive oil with the garlic until the onion looks transparent, a couple of minutes

- Add the uncooked rice, this should also take a couple of minutes and look transparent too

- Add the parsnip and carrots, cook off for a couple of minutes then start adding the stock

- Ladle in the stock to allow the rice and vegetables to cook in a little of the liquid, adding more as ingredients begin to dry, this should take around 20 minutes and by then everything should be cooked

- Just towards the end add the fresh coriander or other herbs

Tips

- If you are feeling in good health and are allowed to have some wine, a glass of dry white added when you add the rice makes a nice change
- This is great if you feel like something filling on a cold winter evening

---

Shepherdless Pie

Serves 4-6

225gm/8oz	Brown lentils (or two 400g/14oz cans of ready cooked, no salt or sugar please)
900g/2lbs	Potatoes, roughly chopped
1 tbsp	Olive oil or coconut oil
3-5 tbsp	Soy milk
225g/8oz	Onions or leeks sliced
1	Clove of garlic, crushed (optional)
115g/4oz	Carrots, diced or sliced
115g/4oz	Parsnips, diced or sliced
225g/8oz	Mushrooms, roughly chopped
3	Sticks celery
2 tbsp	Tomato puree
225gms/8oz	Chopped tomatoes fresh or tinned
1 tbsp	Tamari sauce
½ tsp	Dried rosemary
1 tsp	Dried oregano

Preparation

- Cook the lentils in stock or water until they are tender (about 20-30 minutes).
- Cook the potatoes in boiling salted water. When tender, drain and mash with the milk to obtain creamy (not sloppy) mashed potatoes. Season to taste.
- Meanwhile, heat a little oil in a pan and sauté the onions, garlic, celery, carrots and parsnips until almost tender. If they are slow in cooking, add a little water, cover and cook until just soft.
- Add the mushrooms and continue to cook until they are softening, then add the lentils, tomatoes, tomato puree, oregano and rosemary and cook for a few more minutes. Season to taste with tamari sauce and black pepper
- Spread out in an ovenproof dish. Cover with mashed potatoes about 2cm thick. Bake at 200C (375F, gas 5) for 30-40 minutes

Tips

- Instead of the Tamari sauce try Tabasco or other hot sauce
- The recipe could also be the base for a pasta sauce, may need to increase the stock
- Use half the amount of potatoes and half celeriac or sweet potato or other root vegetable

Trisha Stewart

Marinated Tofu - griddle to perfection or even BBQ'd

Serves 4

450gms/1lb	Tofu cut in 8 slices
5tbsp	Tamari
2	Limes, juiced, or lemons
2tsp	Fresh ginger root, chopped or grated
1-2	Cloves garlic, crushed
1tbs	Good rounded one of fresh chopped coriander, reserve a few leaves for decoration
	Olive oil to ensure this does not stick to the pan when griddling/bbq'ing

Preparation

- In a small bowl mix together the tamari, lime/lemon juice, ginger, garlic and coriander, set aside
- Place the sliced tofu in a ceramic dish, not overlapping so large enough to lay side by side
- Put the marinade over the tofu, cover the dish and leave for about 4 hours or overnight if that works well for you
- Brush the griddle pan with olive oil
- Take the tofu out of the marinade, reserving the marinade for later
- Grill the Tofu on both sides for about 2 mins

Tips

- This is not a meal in itself, but served with a stir fry of vegetables using the marinade as stock would make this delicious, add wild rice to the side and you have a complete meal
- Use the tofu in a soup or casserole with other vegetables

Thai Style Tofu

Serves 4-6

2	Sweet red chillies seeded and chopped
1	Lemon grass stalk chopped
1 inch	Piece of ginger root, peeled and chopped finely
2	Kaffir Lime Leaves
1	Bunch fresh coriander (cilantro)
1 tsp	Ground coriander
1	Pack of Tofu, (plain, smoked or herb) cubed or sliced (or use the marinated recipe from the book
400ml14fl oz	Coconut milk

Preparation

- Put all the above ingredients (except the Tofu) into a food processor or use a pestle and mortar and blend

- Add 400ml of coconut milk to the above and mix together

- Pour in a frying or sauté pan and add the Tofu and simmer so that the ingredients can come together in flavor, about 20 minutes or more if preferred.

Tips

- You can use this sauce as a marinade, just blend the sauce, cube the tofu and leave to marinate together – when ready to eat just heat through

- Serve with rice or other grain and wilted spinach

Spicy, Saucy Chickpeas

Serves 4

450gm/1lb	Dried chickpeas (soaked overnight)
2/3tbsp	Olive oil or sesame oil
115g/4oz	Onions, diced
2	Garlic cloves, crushed or chopped finely
2	Small red chillies finely chopped
1	Small red pepper, deseeded and chopped up
115g/4oz	Carrot, finely diced
2	Sticks of celery, de-strung and finely diced
300ml/12fl oz	Fresh vegetable stock or a good yeast free swiss bouillon
400g/14oz	Tin of chopped tomatoes or fresh diced
2	Large tablespoons fresh coriander plus extra for garnish

Preparation

- Place the chickpeas in a large pan of water and bring to a boil, boil rapidly for 10-15 minutes removing any froth, turn down and simmer for about an hour until they are soft but not broken up.
- Heat the oil in a large sauté or frying pan, put the onion, garlic and chillies in to cook off for 2-3 minutes
- Add the celery, carrots and pepper to the pan and cook off for about 5 minutes
- Pour in the stock, bring to the boil, turn down and simmer for around 15 minutes until vegetables are cooked
- Add the cooked chickpeas, coriander and tomatoes and cook off without the lid on the pan until you have a thick saucy consistency (not mush). You may need to stir, but don't over stir and break everything up!

Tips

- Serve with quinoa or wholegrain rice or wild rice or even rice pasta, and a green salad garnish - perfect!
- You can ring the changes with different vegetables; make it spicier by adding more chilli or cayenne pepper if you want it hot.
- Use different beans such as pinto or haricot or a mix - this dish could work in several different ways.
- Use leftovers to stuff peppers, potatoes or aubergine/eggplant - delicious!

Trisha Stewart

Saucy Roasted Squash

Serves 4

1	Large Butternut Squash or a couple of small ones (less seeds in the smaller ones which is good)
1 tbsp	Olive oil
2	Small fresh red chillies, finely chopped
1	Clove of garlic, crushed
1"	Piece of fresh root ginger finely chopped
1 tbsp	Each peanut butter and tahini (preferably your own fresh made, see recipes)
1 tbsp	Maple syrup or agave nectar
400ml/14oz	Coconut milk
	Handful fresh basil leaves, coarsely chopped

Preparation

- Slice the butternut squash in half lengthways and de-seed and turn over onto the cut side and slice into semi circles
- Lay out on an oiled baking tray, sprinkle a little pure sea salt and a sprinkle of olive oil
- Roast them off in the oven

Make the sauce while that is cooking:

- Heat the oil in a large frying/sauté pan, add onions, garlic, ginger and chillies and sweat off for around 2 minutes
- Add the peanut butter and Tahini and mix through
- Add the coconut milk and simmer for around 10 minutes

- Add in the basil and then remove from the heat
- Pour over the roasted squash (make sure there is no excess oil in the dish of squash)

Tips

- Serve this dish with rice pasta, quinoa or wild rice
- Use any variety of squash
- Add a mixed green salad and some grated beetroot/beets and carrot
- I personally don't like the skin of the butternut squash so just discard if you don't like it either

---

Bolognese Sauce

Serves 4-6

170g/6oz/1cup	Finely chopped onion
2	Cloves garlic, crushed
1"	Piece of fresh root ginger sliced thinly or grated
½ tsp	Cinnamon
1 tbsp	Olive oil or coconut oil
85g/3oz/ ¾ cup	Walnut pieces (toast in a dry frying pan if liked)
300g/12oz/1.5cups	Chopped tomatoes (fresh or tinned)
2 tbsp	Sun dried tomato puree
2 tbsp	Tamari
1	Medium aubergine/eggplant (do not buy large ones as they are usually very seedy and bitter) cut into small cubes or large dice
300ml/10fl oz	Vegetable stock (yeast free) if you are in good health you can substitute half of the liquid for some red wine!

| 1 | Small bunch each of basil and oregano (chopped) |

Preparation

- Put the oil in a pan and sauté off the onions, garlic, ginger and cinnamon, cook until the onions look a little transparent, do not burn
- Add the aubergine/eggplant, cook for a few minutes
- Add the mushrooms and cook for a further five minutes
- Add the remaining ingredients, bring to the boil, turn down and simmer for about 30 minutes, you may need to stir a couple of times.
- At this stage you can choose to blend all of it, half of it or none of it. Choose the texture you want.

Tips

- Serve this with rice pasta or corn pasta
- Use different vegetables from time to time

Red Chilli

Serves 4-6

225g/8oz	Dried red kidney beans (soaked overnight)
2	Medium sized onions, sliced
2	Sticks of celery
2-3	Cloves of garlic, crushed

1	Red pepper, sliced
2-3	Fresh red chillies, de-seeded and chopped finely
400g/14oz	Chopped tomatoes (fresh or tinned)
4 tbsp	Sun dried tomato paste (or plain)
2tsp	Each cumin and coriander seed (ground)
2tsp	Paprika
2tsp	Oregano
1 tbsp	Olive oil or coconut oil

Preparation

- Drain the soaked beans and put in a pan, bring to a boil. Boil fast for 10-15 minutes, skim off any froth, turn down and simmer for 1.5 hours or until just cooked (just firm when pressed together between thumb and finger)
- Heat the oil in a pan, sauté off the onions, garlic for a few minutes
- Add the celery and continue cooking for 1 minute
- Add the peppers, coriander, cumin cook for a further 2 minutes
- Add the chillies and oregano, chopped tomatoes and tomato puree
- Add the beans and paprika and continue to cook for a further 5 -10 minutes (at this stage you can turn the heat right down, put the lid on a leave for a while.

Tips

- Use as many chillies as you like, if you want it hotter add more

Easy Sauté Tofu, Vegetable and Cashew Nuts

Serves 4

300g/10oz	Tofu, cubed
1	Large onion sliced
1	Garlic clove diced
1 inch	Piece of ginger root diced or grated
2	Fresh sweet chillies, de-seeded and chopped finely
	A mix of thinly sliced vegetables such as carrot, green or red peppers, celery, zucchini/courgette, mange tout or fresh peas (any you fancy)
110g/4oz	Cashew Nuts

Preparation

- Heat a small amount of olive oil in a wok or large frying pan
- Add tofu and lightly fry till golden brown, then remove.
- Add the onion and garlic, chili and ginger, sauté for a few minutes
- Put in a mixture of thinly sliced carrots, green pepper, ginger, celery etc and sauté for 1 min to mix flavors
- Add some cashews
- Add a little yeast free stock; put in the tofu and sauté all vegetables until they are as soft as you would like them.

Celeriac and Bean Cakes

Serves 2-4

400g/14oz	Each celeriac and potato
1	Onion, diced
1"	Piece of fresh ginger root, grated
1	Clove of garlic, crushed
½ tsp	Each ground coriander, cumin, cinnamon, chili
2 tsp	Tamari sauce
400g/14oz	Cooked adzuki beans
2 tsp	Olive oil or coconut oil

Preparation

- Peel and cut the potato and celeriac into similar sizes and put in a pan of water, bring to a boil, turn down and simmer until tender, remove from the heat and put into a colander to drain off
- Put the oil into a pan and sauté the onion, garlic and ginger for a few minutes until soft but not browned
- Add the spices and cook off for about five minutes, do not have the heat to high
- Put the potato, celeriac and spices into a bowl and add the beans and tamari sauce
- Mix it all together and then form into individual cakes
- Then add a little oil to a frying pan and cook the cakes till browned or put under the grill

Tips

- You can make any vegetable cakes in this way
- Vary the type of vegetables and beans used
- Ring the changes with the spices and oils
- Use left-over vegetables and potatoes in this way - we call them Bubble and Squeak cakes in the UK or at least in Devon!
- Serve on their own for breakfast or with a salad for lunch
- Sprout the adzuki beans and add them to the rest of the ingredients

---

Baked Sweet Potato

Serves 2

2	Large sweet potatoes (one for each person)
1	Onion, diced
1 tsp	Olive oil or coconut oil
½ tsp	Each ground coriander and cumin
6	Small button mushrooms cut into quarters
1 tsp	Tamari sauce
1 tsp	Oregano

Preparation

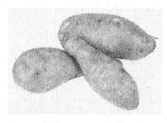

- Heat oven to 190c/375f/gas 5
- Wash over the potatoes and rub a little oil into the skins (minimal), place on a baking tray and cook for about 45-60 minutes till soft inside

- Heat the oil in a pan and sweat off the onion for a few minutes until soft
- Add the mushrooms and spices to the pan and cook for another few minutes
- Add in the tamari sauce and oregano
- Remove pan from heat
- Cut each potato carefully in half, try and get the flesh out in little cubes or rounds and place in a bowl
- Add the onion mixture to this and gently mix together
- Put the mix back into the potato skins and bake off in the oven till nicely browned or put under the grill

Tips

- Vary the types of potato
- Use any other vegetable instead of mushrooms such as diced peppers and celery
- Eat as a lunch dish with a green salad or even for breakfast

---

Tofu and Pineapple Stir Fry

Serves 4

1	Fresh pineapple, peeled and cut into chunks
2	Fresh red Chili (de-seeded)
2	Clove of garlic
1"	Piece of fresh root ginger - grated or sliced
3tbsp	Each tamari sauce, apple cider vinegar
1 ½ tsp	Cornflour/corn starch
1 pack	Tofu cut into small cubes
2tsp	Olive oil or coconut oil
2	Leeks sliced across thinly

1	Red pepper de-seeded and sliced
2	Carrot cut into matchsticks
1	Courgette/zuchinni cut diagonally
20	Mange tout
1	Large handful of bean sprouts
1	Large handful of Chinese leaves
1	Handful of fresh coriander

Preparation

- Put the first 6 ingredients into a blender and whizz up, set aside
- Put the tofu under the grill and toast for a few minutes
- Heat the oil in a pan and add the leeks, red pepper and carrot and cook off for 5-10 minutes
- Add the rest of the vegetables and tofu and stir fry for 3-5 minutes
- Add the blended ingredients to the pan and bring to bubbling point for 3 minutes

Tips

- Serve alone or with wild rice or wholegrain rice

Shitake Steaks (these can be used in various ways, see Tip)

Serves 4

(depending on what you do with it)

20	Dried Shitake mushrooms (soaked in a covered bowl of cold water, overnight)
3tbsp	Sunflower or olive oil
2 tbsp	Tamari sauce
1 tbsp	Toasted sesame oil

Preparation

- Drain the shitake reserving 120ml/4 fl oz of the liquid – pick the mushrooms out by hand and take the liquid from the top of the bowl as these mushrooms can be very gritty
- Remove and throw away the stalks
- Heat the sunflower or olive oil in a wok or frying pan and stir fry the mushrooms for 5 minutes on a fairly high heat, stirring all the time.
- Reduce heat to the lowest setting and add the liquid and tamari sauce, cook the mushrooms until the pan is almost dry, add the toasted sesame oil and remove from the heat.
- Leave to cool

Tips

- Slice into thin strips and add to 400g/14oz of cooked wholegrain basmati rice, add chopped chives and put into individual bowls and serve. Great as a lunch box special.

- Serve with marinated tofu or as a side dish to any of the other recipes.
- Serve on a bed of leaves as a starter.

Creamy Mushroom Stroganoff

Serves 4

450g/1lb	Mushrooms (button or small firm ones), sliced
2 tbsp	Olive, sunflower or coconut oil
1-2	Cloves of garlic, crushed
1	Onion, diced
425ml/ ¾ pt	Fresh vegetable stock of yeast free bouillon
350g/ ¾ lb	Silken tofu
Pinch	Sea salt
1 tsp	Grainy mustard
Pinch	Fresh ground black pepper

Preparation

- Heat the oil in a frying pan or wok and fry off the mushrooms till they are tender, just a few minutes
- Add the garlic and onion and cook off for a further 2 minutes
- Add the cornflour/corn starch. Stir well and slowly add the stock to avoid a lumpy sauce
- Put the tofu and mustard in a blender/liquidizer with a little water at a time; try to make around 600ml/1 pt of the sauce. Whizz to a nice a creamy consistency
- Add to the mushroom mix and heat through.

Tips

- Be careful about the liquids in both the mushroom mix and the tofu blend as mushrooms can be a little watery so you may need less.
- Serve with wholegrain basmati rice, quinoa or rice pasta.
- Include a lovely green salad.

Stuffed Peppers

Serves 4

4	Red, yellow or green peppers or a mix
225g/8oz	Tofu
1	Medium onion, diced
2	Cloves of garlic, crushed
2	Small – medium tomatoes, diced
1	Small courgette/zuchinni, diced
3 tbsp	Almonds coarsely chopped and toasted in a dry fry pan
¼ tsp	Ground cinnamon
½ tsp	Ground cumin
Pinch	Cayenne pepper
Pinch	Sea salt
Splash	Tabasco or Jalapeno Sauce
6fl oz/200ml	Tomato juice
2 tbsp	Chopped fresh coriander

Preparation

- Pre-heat the oven to 180c/350f/gas 4

- Cut the top off the peppers, keeping the stalk intact, remove the seeds and any white flesh
- Place the peppers cut side down and the lids on a lightly oiled baking sheet, rub a little oil into the skin
- Bake for 10-15 minutes just to give them some cooking time as they will go back into the oven shortly
- Meanwhile, heat the oil in a frying pan and sauté the onions, garlic, courgette/zuchinni, cumin and cayenne pepper for about 5 minutes until onion is softened
- Add the tomatoes and cook off for about 5 minutes
- Roughly crumble the tofu and add to the mix with 3 parts of the almonds and simmer for 5 more minutes
- Remove the peppers from the oven and cool so that you can handle them
- Stuff the peppers with the mix, pressing the mix in gently so as not to break the sides of the pepper
- Pour the tomato juice over the top of each with a splash of tabasco or other hot sauce if liked and put the lids of the peppers on top, you may cover lightly with foil to avoid burning
- Cook off for around 30-40 minutes
- Remove from the oven and garnish with the rest of the almonds and coriander

Tips

- These are delicious with the hot pepper sauce (see recipe section)
- Served with wholegrain basmati or wild rice
- Served with a large green salad

Potato Wedges

Serves 4

6	White potatoes cut into quarters (less or more depending on size of potato)
1 tbsp	Olive oil or coconut oil
Pinch	Sea salt
Pinch	Dried herbs such as thyme, rosemary, sage, basil – anything you fancy

Preparation

- Pre-heat the oven to 220c/425f/gas 6

- Put the oil, salt and herbs into a plastic food bag

- Add the potatoes and shake till they are coated in the oil and herbs

- Take out of bag and spread on an oven tray

- Cook for around 25 minutes until nice and crispy but cooked through

Tips

- Serve with the Slaw from the recipe section
- Add a green salad and vegan mayo (from the recipe section)
- Use sweet potatoes but reduce the cooking time

Stuffed Mushrooms

Serves 4

(1 large mushroom per person)

4	Large, flat, open mushrooms
100g/4oz	Pitted olives
1-2	Cloves of garlic
100g/4oz	Walnuts, cashews or other nuts
1 tbsp	Fresh chopped parsley or other herb

Preparation

- Preheat oven to 190c/375f/gas 5

- Remove the stalks from the mushrooms and place in a blender with the olives and walnuts and garlic; whizz to a paste and set aside

- Put the mushrooms on a lightly oiled baking tray and stuff the mixture into each one, taking care to spread to the edges

- Bake off for around 20 - 25 minutes until cooked

Tips

- Have these as a starter on a bed of raw spinach
- Put alongside the marinated tofu or other dish as a side dish

Kedgeree with a Twist

Serves 4

60g/2oz	Dried lentils (red, brown or green) rinsed and picked over for any little stones
1	Bay leaf or bouquet garni bundle
225/8oz	Wholegrain basmati rice
4	Cloves
2 tbsp	Olive or coconut oil
1 tsp	Creole Spice Mix (see recipe)
Bunch	Parsley or coriander, chopped

Preparation

- Get two pans and place the rice and cloves in one and the lentils and bay leaf in the other and cover with cold water, bring to a boil, turn down and simmer for 20 minutes or so until they are cooked (with the lid on)

- Heat the oil in a pan and cook off the spices for a minute

- Drain the rice and lentils removing the cloves and bay leaf and stir into the spice mix

- Cook off for a couple of minutes stirring to coat the grains

Tips

- Great for breakfast, lunch or dinner or to prepare for exercise
- Add one or two of the salads for a great meal

Curry Paste, Sauce, Accompaniments

How many different curries do you
really need?

The key to any curry is the right
kind of base which of course is the
choice of spices – do you want it
hot or mild, medium or Thai style.

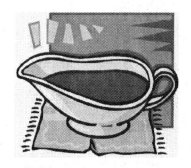

I risk being shot by any true native
or curry fan – but let me say here I
totally respect their tradition but
for most of us all we want is a tasty spicy dish – it is, after all,
a spicy stew whatever you put in it or call it.

Please use fresh, organic ingredients where possible, DO NOT
use the old spices that have been kicking about in the back of
the cupboard for years, their lovely pungent smell and taste
will have long gone.

I am listing four different styles of curry paste/sauce; all you
need do is add your vegetables, lentils beans, tofu or
whatever. So, for aubergine/eggplant madras style, you just
choose the madras sauce or for chickpea korma style you
choose the mild korma style or a vegetable vindaloo, you got
it! vindaloo sauce!

If you don't have all the ingredients for one sauce make a mix
just remember it's about how it tastes to you and the people
that are going to eat it!

Healthy Bunch Cook Book

The heat comes from the chillies or chilli powder or cayenne in the main so the more of those you add the hotter it will be.

Mild Korma Style
---

3 tsps	Ground coriander
1.5 tsp	Ground chilli powder
1 tsp	Each fennel and cumin seeds
½ tsp	Ground turmeric
½ inch	Fresh ginger root
2	Large cloves of garlic
200ml/7fl oz	Coconut milk
2 tbsp	Coconut oil
½ tsp	Each fenugreek and fennel seeds
2 inch	Cinnamon stick
225g/8oz	Onions, sliced
225g/8oz	Tomatoes, chopped
Little	Sea salt
½	Juice of fresh lime

Directions

1. Put the first six ingredients into a blender with 2 tbsp water and puree – set aside.
2. Heat the oil in a pan and sauté off the fenugreek and fennel seeds and the cinnamon for a few seconds till you hear the seeds popping.
3. Add the onion and sauté for a few minutes until transparent.
4. Add the spice mix (first six ingredients that you have pureed (if it sticks to the pan add a few drops of water.
5. Add the tomatoes and sauté for 2-3 minutes *(if you are going to freeze the sauce, stop here) (if you are going to carry on with the cooking, this is also where you add*

your vegetables, lentils, beans, tofu or whatever you are going to put into the curry).

6. Add 300ml/½ pt warm water with a little salt. Bring to a boil and turn down immediately. Simmer for around 20 minutes until everything is cooked to your liking.
7. Add the coconut milk and lime juice. Bring back to the boil and then turn off the heat.

Tips

- Keep the first four ingredients ready mixed in a little jar and label "mild curry spices"
- Double, treble or more of this recipe to step 5 then all you have to do is take out what you need and add step 6 and 7.
- You can freeze the whole thing but I find the vegetables go soggy when frozen, but that may not bother you.
- At step 5 you can put the ingredients into the refrigerator as this will keep for 4/5 days.
- If you want this a little hotter add in more chilli powder or some fresh chilli at step 1.

Medium Madras Style

8-12	Dried red whole chillies (soaked in water for 10 minutes to soften)
3 tsps	Each ground paprika and coriander
4	Peppercorns
2	Bay leaves
4"/10cm	Cinnamon stick
6	Whole cloves
1 tsp	Each poppy and cumin seeds
½ tsp	Fennel seeds

1"/2.5cm	Piece of fresh ginger root
6	Large cloves of garlic
2 tbsp	Coconut oil
2	Large onions, sliced
4	Large tomatoes, chopped
200ml/7 fl oz	Coconut milk

Directions

1. Grind/blend together the first 10 ingredients, adding a little water to make a paste consistency
2. Heat the oil in a pan and sweat off the onions, browning slightly
3. Add the paste you have made and cook for 10-15 minutes stirring in around 3tbsp of water to keep from drying out
4. Add the chopped tomatoes and cook for around 5 minutes *(if you are going to freeze, stop here)*
5. Put your choice of vegetables, lentils, tofu, beans (make sure these are cooked if dried or tinned if not)
6. Add 200ml/7 fl oz of water , bring back to a boil and simmer the whole dish for around 20 minutes until everything is cooked
7. Add the coconut milk and bring back to a boil, turn off the heat and let it sit for a minute

Tips

- Take the first 8 dried ingredients and put into a jar and store as "madras style spice mix"
- If you are going to freeze this take it to step 4 make sure you double up or more to save time
- You can freeze the whole thing but I find the vegetables go soggy when frozen, but that may not bother you
- At step 5 you can put the ingredients into the refrigerator as this will keep for 4/5 days

Hot Vindaloo Style

6	Cloves
5cm/2"	Cinnamon stick
10	Peppercorns
¼	Star anise
1 tsp	Poppy seeds
1 tsp	Cumin seeds
5cm/2"	Fresh ginger root
6	Large cloves of garlic
15-20	Whole red dried chilies (soaked in water for 10 minutes to soften)
1 tbsp	Tamarind pulp (or juice of 1 lime)
4tsps	Apple cider vinegar
1tbsp	Coconut oil
3	Medium/large onions, sliced
15	Curry leaves

Directions

1. Blend the first 11 ingredients, set aside
2. Heat the oil in a pan and sauté off the onions for 10 – 15 minutes (do not burn)
3. Add the blended ingredients and cook for 5 minutes, stirring and adding a little water to ensure it does not dry out
4. Put your choice of vegetables, cooked beans, lentils, tofu into the mixture and cook off for 10 minutes
5. Add 400ml/14 fl oz water, sometimes more or less depending on the type of vegetables you are using – for instance root vegetables can absorb more than peppers and mushrooms.

6. Bring to the boil, turn down and simmer until everything is cooked to your liking – around 20-25 minutes

Tips

- At step 3, the ingredients will keep in the refrigerator for 4/5 days
- Double or triple the ingredients to step 3 if you are going to freeze, this will save time
- If you are going to freeze this do it at step 3 also, as I have said before I find the other ingredients make it too soggy after freezing, but that is just my opinion

---

Thai Style

2	Sweet red chilies seeded and chopped
1	Lemon grass stalk chopped
1 inch	Piece of ginger root, peeled and chopped finely
2	Kaffir Lime Leaves
2	Cloves of garlic
1 bunch	Fresh coriander (cilantro) chopped finely
400ml/14 fl oz	Coconut milk
2	Medium onions, sliced
1 tbsp	Coconut oil

Directions

1. Blend the first five ingredients, set aside
2. Heat the oil in a pan and sauté the onions for 5-10 minutes until soft
3. Add the coconut milk and coriander and bring to a boil, turn off the heat and allow to sit for a while. *(if you*

are going to use the sauce immediately, now is the time to add your chosen ingredients and cook on for about 20-25 minutes)

Tips

- Tofu works well here, see recipe for marinated tofu
- Cooked beans or legumes work well here too, especially chickpeas
- Add some red peppers for a great color and taste or some julienne carrots and fresh peas
- Longer cooking root vegetables do not work so well in this sauce unless you pre-cook them
- Coarsely chop some peanuts or almonds and scatter through the sauce

Red Lentil Dhal

1 tsp	Garlic, crushed
1 tsp	Each fresh chilli and ginger, finely chopped and mixed
2 tsp	Powdered turmeric
1 tsp	Each garam masala and ground coriander
2 tbsp	Fresh coriander, finely chopped
1	Cinnamon stick
1 tsp	Mustard
1 large	Tomato, diced finely
1 medium	Onion, diced finely
2 sticks	Celery, diced finely
1tbsp	Olive oil or coconut oil
600ml/20fl oz	Filtered water
225gms/8oz	Red lentils, washed well

Preparation

- Heat the oil in a saucepan with a thick base
- Add the garlic, chilli, ginger and spices (except fresh coriander), herbs, mustard, tomato, onion and celery.
- Fry for about 10 minutes until well blended.
- Add water and bring to a boil
- Stir in the lentils and cook on a low heat for about half an hour, until the lentils are soft, stirring occasionally. Take off the heat and stir in the fresh coriander.

Tips

- You may need to add a little stock or water if the dhal becomes dry.
- If you have time place a couple of bulbs of garlic in the oven and roast for half an hour, take out and press the juicy roasted garlic and add to the dhal
- Sprinkle some chopped almonds on top
- This is a good side dish for a vegetable curry

Bombay Potatoes

4	Medium sized sweet potatoes (cut into cubes)
1 tsp	Ground turmeric
½ tsp	Cumin
1	Lemon, juice and zest
2	Cloves of garlic
1 tbsp	Chopped fresh coriander
1	Medium sized red pepper (de-seeded and chopped)
1"	Piece of fresh root ginger thinly sliced

4	Large tomatoes (coarsely chopped)
1	Very large handful of spinach

Directions

- Place the cubed potatoes in a large bowl
- Blend the turmeric, cumin, lemon juice, ginger and garlic
- Rub the blended mix all over the potatoes with your clean hands
- Place in a lightly oiled baking tray and add the tomatoes
- Cook in a pre-heated oven 200c/400f/gas6 for around 20-30- minutes until potato is cooked, take care this does not burn, you may need to add a little water to the pan
- 5 minutes before the end of cooking throw in the spinach and mix around the potatoes and cook for a further 5 minutes

Tips

- This works with white potatoes but you may need to adjust the cooking time
- The whole thing can be cooked in a large shallow pan on the stove. You may need to add a little water to the cooking.
- Serve with any curry, dhal or on its own

Rice

I prefer you to use wholegrain basmati rice, these recipes all take a little longer to cook because of this. Wild rice makes a nice change too.

Plain Boiled Rice

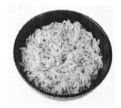

There are several ways to cook rice, a rice boiler is a great idea but I use a pan, bring the water to the boil add in the rice, bring back to the boil and simmer with the lid on till cooked, around 20 minutes, the rice should be cooked and the water absorbed. If the grains don't separate it has been cooked too long, you should just be able to gently squeeze the grain between finger and thumb.

Cook up enough for several days as you can always use it in the lunch boxes. Keep refrigerated.

Tips

- A rule of thumb for the amount of rice to water is 1 part rice to 1 1/3 part water - enough rice for two people is 200g/7oz rice and 265ml/9 ½ fl oz water
- For fragrant rice add ½" cinnamon stick, whole bay leaf, 1 cardamom clove, 1 clove, if you can wrap these in a little muslin and put this in with the cooking water, great, if not put the individual items in and fish them out before serving.

- For yellow rice add a pinch of turmeric to boiling water.
- For saffron rice, soak a few strands of saffron in three tbsp of boiling water for 30 minutes, add to the cooked rice.

Wholegrain Basmati Pilaf

Serves 4

1 tbsp	Cardamom Seeds
1 inch	Cinnamon stick
1 tsp	Each cumin seeds, whole cloves, peppercorns
1/3	Whole nutmeg
1 tsp	Black mustard seeds (yellow if you can't get them)
1	Medium onion, sliced
2	cloves garlic
1 inch	Piece of fresh ginger
200g/7oz	Basmati rice
225g/8oz	Mushrooms
1 tsp	Ground coriander
1tbsp	Olive oil or coconut oil
6fl oz/ ¾ cup	Filtered water or yeast free vegetable stock

Directions

- Grind the first four ingredients in a pestle and mortar or coffee grinder, set aside
- Heat the oil in a shallow pan and add the mustard seeds, onions, garlic and ginger and sauté for around 5-

10 minutes, don't allow anything to burn adding a little water if necessary
- Stir in the rice and cook off for a few minutes
- Add the mushrooms and ground spices that you have set aside and cook for 1 minute
- Add the water slowly, stirring and then bring to a boil, turn down to simmer for around 20-25 minutes until rice is cooked and water has been absorbed.
- Remove from the heat and let stand for a few minutes

Tips

- Add a little more water if necessary to ensure everything is cooked
- Ring the changes with other vegetables such as peas, courgette/zucchini, peppers
- Add in some pine nuts, almonds or other chopped nuts

Fried Rice

170g/6oz	Wholegrain basmati rice
14fl oz/1 ¾ cups	Filtered water
¼ tsp	Turmeric
1	Courgette/zucchini, red pepper, carrot, cut into sticks or julienned
4	Small red or white onions
6	Medium mushrooms
1½ tsp	Sesame oil
½ tsp	Mirin (rice wine)
1 tbsp	Tamari sauce

Directions

- Cook the rice by putting the water into a pan and bringing to a boil, add the rice, bring back to a boil, turn down and simmer till cooked, around 20 minutes. Keep the lid on and don't stir. The water should be absorbed and the rice cooked.
- Whilst the rice is cooking, heat half the oil in a shallow pan and put in the mushrooms and courgette/zucchini, cook off for 2-3 minutes, set aside, don't overcook as these will go soggy
- Heat the oil in a shallow pan or a wok and add the onion and turmeric, cook for 5 minutes
- Add the rice and continue cooking for a few minutes.
- Add the tamari sauce and mirin and the vegetables to the rice toss, gently heat for a minute to make sure everything is hot and then serve.

Tips

- Leave to cool and have a great lunchbox filler.
- Vary the vegetables and have carrots, peas and peppers.
- Add in some parsley or coriander, freshly chopped.

Raita relish, dip or condiment

200m/l7 fl oz	Soy yogurt
1/8 tsp	Cumin powder
Pinch	Paprika
4" piece	Cucumber finely diced
1 tbsp	Finely crushed coriander leaves

- Whisk the yogurt
- Add the other ingredients
- Garnish with fresh coriander

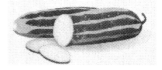

Tips

You can make another 5 different ones by changing the recipe to the following

- finely diced tomato
- onion
- cooked potato
- blanched shredded spinach
- Fresh red chili de-seeded and shredded thinly

Notes on curry section:

- You will find other spicy dishes in the book but I wanted you to try and get a quick fix curry without resorting to jars and packets from the supermarket.
- There are plenty more ways to have a curry but most of them have too much dairy, sugar and far too much oil so these will certainly keep the taste buds tingling without too many calories

Afters / Desserts

This is going to be a fairly small chapter -
due to the fact that I am avoiding the use
of wheat, dairy, sugar and yeast - you can
get plenty of those recipes anywhere!

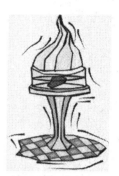

I have put together some really quick
sweet fixes and a few everyday puddings
that will keep you satisfied and have your
taste buds tingling.

Please be aware, some of the recipes have dried fruit which
has a higher sugar content than fresh, therefore higher in
calories - also I am using maple syrup in some - again increasing
the calorie load, you need to watch the GI if you are diabetic
or have sugar handling problems.

Remember also, topping with cream or ice cream from the
recipes is increasing the content of natural sugars from the
dried fruit and maple syrup; also the protein and fats from the
nuts. If you are overweight then you really need to avoid this
section altogether or just opt for the fruit salads in the
breakfast section.

Ice Cream - yes - real ice cream without all the preservatives,
colorings and other junk.

Nut Ice Cream

Serves 2 unless you are greedy!

225g/8oz	Nut butter* (see recipe)
120ml/4fl oz	Maple syrup
115g/4oz	Coarsely chopped almonds
1 tsp	Almond Essence

Directions

- Put all the ingredients into a bowl or blender and mix thoroughly
- Put into little serving pots or even ice cube trays and freeze

Tips

- Try adding some carob powder or vanilla essence for a different taste
- Vary the type of nuts you use
- Try some grated coconut in the mix
- BE AWARE this is very high in calories

Banana Ice Cream

Serves 2

4	Ready frozen bananas
250ml/8fl oz	Freshly squeezed orange juice
115g/4oz	Cashew nuts
150g/5oz	Soft dates, preferably soaked in warm water for a couple of hours

Directions

- Blend and chill for twenty minutes

Tips

- Use any frozen fruit, berries, mango or kiwi
- Vary the type of nuts
- Add in some carob
- Add in some coconut
- Make this whatever you want it to be

Berry Dream

Serves 2

300g/10oz	Berries
2 tbsp	Finely chopped dates
300ml/10fl oz	Cream (see recipe)

Directions

- Whip the ingredients together and serve in nice tall glasses with a sprinkling of toasted nuts and seeds

Tips

- Use any fruit for this, the idea is to make a creamy mouse like desert - anything goes

---

Baked Apple Crumble

Serves 4

450g/1 lb	Naturally sweet eating apples
1	Lemon freshly squeezed
2fl oz	Apple juice
115g/4oz	Pure vegan margarine
60g/2oz	Oats
85g/3oz	Rice flour
60g/2oz	Millet flakes
1 tsp	Ground cinnamon

Directions

- Slice the apples and place in a lightly oiled oven proof dish, sprinkle the lemon juice over, add the apple juice
- Put the rest of the ingredients into a bowl and "rub" the margarine in with your fingertips so that you get a crumbly type of mix
- Sprinkle the crumble topping over the apples and bake for around 30-40 minutes in an oven 350f/180c Gas 4

Tips

- Choose any fruit
- Add some grated coconut to the crumble mix
- Use nutmeg instead of cinnamon
- Top with one of the cream or ice cream recipes

Crunchy Nut Rice Pudding

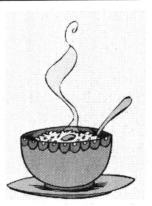

Serves 4-6

600g/21 oz	Pre-cooked short grain brown rice (pudding rice)
600ml/20 fl oz	Rice or nut milk
1	Orange, juiced and grated rind
115g/4 oz	Sultanas/raisins
1 tbsp	Maple syrup (could be omitted)
1 tbsp	Grated coconut
115g/4 oz	Chopped nuts
1 tsp	Nutmeg

Directions

- Put the pre-cooked rice and milk into a pan and bring to the boil, reduce heat and simmer on low for around 10-15 mins
- Add the sultanas/raisins, orange juice and rind and simmer for a minute

- Add the nuts and maple syrup and turn off the heat and let this sit for a couple of minutes
- Put into a serving bowl or individual bowls and sprinkle with nutmeg

Tips

- Vary the nuts
- Use 1 tsp agave nectar instead of the maple syrup
- Choose some finely chopped dates instead of the sultanas/raisins
- Top with cream from the recipes in book

Baked Fresh Figs

2	Fresh figs per person (more if you like)
1	Orange, juice and grated rind
1 tbsp	Olive oil or sesame oil
1	Handful of pistachio nuts

Directions

- Lightly oil a baking dish and place the figs in the dish
- Drizzle with a little oil
- Sprinkle over the pistachio nuts
- Pour over the orange juice and rind
- Bake in a preheated oven180c/350f/Gas 4, for 15-20 minutes (they only really have to be heated through)

Tips

- Top with cream from the recipes

Stuffed Apples

1	Apple per person
1 tsp	Finely chopped nuts per person
1 tsp	Tahini per person
1 tsp	Sultanas/raisins per person

Directions

- Take the core from the apple
- Put the rest of the ingredients in a bowl and mix well
- Stuff into the centre of the apple
- Put in a lightly oiled baking dish and bake off for 20-30 minutes at 180c/350f/Gas4

Tips

- Top with a cream or ice cream from the recipes

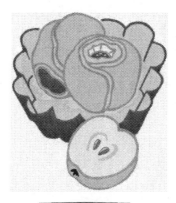

Cooking and prep tips

This list is by no means extensive but it does cover the ingredients you are using throughout the book. Starting with rice as I feel it is one of the most versatile and useful ingredients in anyone's diet.

There will be further information on my website regarding health matters and the use of whole grains and many other food products. I just want to get you preparing food, both raw and cooked and enjoying it all without too much "ado".

The following two types of rice are those I would recommend for your immediate work towards becoming one of the Healthy Bunch

- Wholegrain Basmati rice is the one of my favorites. It takes longer to cook than the white refined, is far more nutritious than white or other rice as it has a slower release of carbohydrates. Use twice the amount of water to rice, bring to a boil and simmer with the lid on until most or all of the water is absorbed.
- Wild Rice is actually an aquatic grass, it is a dramatic brown/black color and is nutty to taste, takes longer than most grains to cook but can be soaked overnight to reduce the time. It is very nutritious as it contains all the essential amino acids and is rich in lysine. Cook as above

Other rice you could use for a change or depending on whether or not you are cooking a paella or risotto could include Jasmine, Red Carmargue, Arborio for risottos, Valencia for Paella.

I have included the use of rice flour in this book it is a great alternative to wheat flour as it is virtually gluten free. You could also use potato flour but this is very starchy and you do not need to use too much. Rice pasta is also a great alternative to wheat pasta. Soy flour is gluten free so also a good alternative to wheat.

How to keep cooked rice or other grain free from bacteria

- Keep a batch over no more than 3 days
- Cook according to which grain you are using and rinse off with cold water, drain and put in the fridge except for the portion you may be using at that meal. This will ensure that when you want to throw a grain dish together you already have the base ingredients.
- Should you wish to refresh and use hot, bring a pan of water to a boil, put the grain in a bring back to a boil for 60 seconds
- You can also sauté the grain if making a risotto the fast way
- Cold rice is always ready for your salad and lunchbox

The benefits of eating whole grains and whole cereals include a slow release of carbohydrate (low GI or GL) low fat, good source of protein, fiber, vitamins and minerals,

Other Grains or cereals

- Oats come in jumbo, rolled, flaked, oatmeal, oat bran for making porridge, oatcakes and pancakes. These are glutinous, not as much as wheat but should be avoided or limited to people with celiac disease.

- Quinoa (Pronounced keen-wah) is a supergrain as it contains all the essential amino acids. Does not take as long as wholegrain rice to cook and doubles in size. As a rule of thumb for one person ½ cup quinoa to 1 cup of water, bring to boil and simmer with the lid on.

- Millet grains, flakes and flour are gluten free. Ideal for porridge or use as a change from rice.
- Buckwheat is not wheat but of the rhubarb family. It is gluten free and comes plain or toasted and is used in pancakes (from buckwheat flour), porridge (Kasha) and Japanese soba noodles.

Legumes

Legumes are a very versatile and nutritious food with a range of shapes and textures. They are an important part of protein in a vegetarian diet as well as fiber, vitamins and minerals, low in fat, low GI/GL and slow release of carbohydrates.

- Red, yellow, green, brown, puy are all lentils. These do not need soaking, wash and pick over as there maybe stones in them
- Red, split lentils have the shortest cooking time and develop into a mush and are very suited to making Dhal or for thickening soups, as are the yellow ones
- Green and brown take longer to cook and retain their shape so are ideal as they can be used for salads, casseroles etc
- Puy lentils keep their shape and also look very nice, are superior in taste and texture and suited to salads because of the way the look and taste but can be used in any dish
- Peas, split, marrow fat are great for adding to soups and casseroles or making "mushy peas" or pease pudding. They need soaking overnight.

Pulses/Beans are an important part of any diet. Packed with protein and fiber, vitamins, minerals and are extremely low in fat/ low GI/GL.

- They are ideal fill up foods when you are on a weight-loss program.
- These do need to be soaked overnight and then cooked. You can buy them in tins but you must choose salt and sugar free but remember anything in a tin will already have been well cooked so not as good as your own but sometimes a necessary standby.
- There are great benefits to sprouting beans (pulses) see sprouting section in book.

To prepare and cook:

- Soak overnight or at least 5-6 hours, remove from the water and rinse, place in a large pan with water and bring to a boil, skim and simmer for 1-2 hours depending on type of bean, check for tenderness (just soft as you press between finger and thumb.
- Do not add salt to the water as this will make them tough but to prevent flatulence add ginger, dill and caraway to the cooking water.
- Here is a list of some of the beans to use, all have an interesting taste and texture, choose your favorites as any one of them will be useful to your eating program.
- Aduki (adzuki), black-eyed, black turtle are often used in oriental cooking, Creole and Indian cooking, but can be used whenever you need beans
- Cannellini, borlotti, butter, haricot, flageolet, and pinto are what I would term as the softer bean, used in European cooking
- Chick peas or Garbanzo are like little nuts with a creamy flavor.

- Kidney well remembered for their use in South American cooking, these keep their shape and look great in salads. They do, however need special care when bringing to a boil. Boil vigorously for 10-15 minutes as they contain a substance that can cause food poisoning. They also require a longer soaking period of about 8-12 hours.
- All of the beans will be a great addition to curry, salads, refried, mashed into a puree. Add full flavors from herbs and spices to enhance the taste.

Soy Bean Products

Tofu or bean curd is exactly what is says, the curd from the milk of the bean. It comes in various textures, shapes and flavors.

This product is high in protein, very low in fat and an excellent alternative to meat.

- Firm is a block of Tofu which can be cubed, sliced and used as kebabs, in salads, stir fry, casserole or mashed and made into burgers, rissoles, patties. This product is very bland and does improve with marinating or you can buy smoked, herbed or deep fried.

Silken Tofu   Has a smoother texture and is ideal for sauces, dips, dressings. A very useful dairy alternative. Keep covered in water and in the fridge for up to one week.

Tempeh   This is made by fermenting cooked soy beans. It has a nuttier taste and if you are missing meat the texture is firmer and it works well in casseroles and pies or marinated and sliced with a sauce

Soy Sauce   Is made by combining crushed soy beans, wheat, salt, water and a yeast based culture called Koji and is left to ferment from 6 months to 3 years. Hence you will pay more for the best quality. Try to buy naturally brewed as there are a lot of chemically prepared products on the market so they ferment faster. The dark sauce is heavier and sweeter whilst the light is thinner and saltier

Tamari   This product is made without the wheat so is gluten free. Can be used in cooking or as a condiment

Miso   Made from cooked soy beans, rice, wheat or barley, salt and water and is left to ferment for about 3 years. You can add it to soups, stock, stir fry and noodle dishes. There are three types, Kome or white miso is the lightest in strength, Mugi is a medium strength and Hacho is dark, rich and thick and has a strong flavor.

- All of the above sauces are very salty in taste so use sparingly.

Soy milk, cream and yogurt are good dairy alternatives. As are rice and nut milks, creams and butters.

Nuts

- Pecan, pine, walnuts, pistachio, macadamia, cashew, almonds, brazils (Brazils are high in saturated fat so take it easy), chestnuts, hazelnuts, coconuts, Always buy as fresh as possible and in small quantities, if buying in shell they should feel heavy for their size, this will indicate freshness.

Coconut contains saturated fats and therefore should be used with caution but it is a great addition to curry. Coconut oil works better for general use as it can withstand a higher cooking temperature without changing its properties.

- Most nuts are high in either mono/poly unsaturated fats. They are packed with protein, vitamins and minerals.

Seeds

- Sesame, Sunflower, Poppy, Pumpkin, Hemp and Linseeds (flax) are all rich with essential fatty acids and protein, vitamins and minerals. You can make seed butter in the same way as nut butter.
- Purchase in small quantities. Dry roasting brings out the flavor. Grinding releases the oils and is the best method for using these nutritious foods.
- Seeds can also be sprouted. And, they are packed with essential fatty acids, protein, vitamins and minerals.

Fruit and Vegetable Kingdom

- Providing energy, fiber, vitamins and minerals, antioxidants, beta-carotene, phytochemicals, bioflavonoids and have fabulous health giving properties.

Roots/Tubers   Root vegetables are comforting and nourishing and popular in winter; leave the outer skins on where possible as this is a great source of natural fiber.

Carrots These are not just a good winter vegetable as we get the summer crops too. Choose the smaller ones as they will be sweeter. Suitable to eat raw, juiced, steamed, stir fried or roasted.

Beetroot/Beets Beetroot/beets can have an "earthy" taste particularly when juiced. They add a fabulous color to salads if grated, used in risottos or soups or roasted, mashed. Take care when washing so the skin does not get damaged as the red color will leach out. Choose firm products do not accept them if the skin is wrinkly they will be old and woody. Beetroot/beets have always been considered a "tonic" to help disorders of the blood including anemia.

Celeriac Similar in flavor to celery. This must be peeled but can be eaten raw, cooked and mashed, baked, steamed or in a soup. Try mashing with other roots to get a blend of flavors. It makes a great topping for vegetable bakes or in sheperdless pie.

Parsnip Sweet tasting and works well roasted, mashed, pureed, grated or I love them with carrots in a risotto. These are best bought after the first frost as it is said the cold converts the starch into sugar enhancing its sweetness. Avoid old or limp products as they will be woody and not at all nice.

Swede/Rutabaga Good raw, steamed, mashed and as a mix with others that mash.

Turnips   These have a slight peppery taste, depending on their size; choose small firm ones. You can Boil, steam, bake, roast or eat raw.

Potatoes   There are far too many to name, all with their distinctive flavor and uses. Do not use potatoes that have green patches. Depending on the type, choose your favorite way of cooking them.

Sweet Potatoes/Yams   Suited to mashing, roasting or roasting. slighter slower release of energy than the white potato.

Jerusalem Artichokes   These are often knobbly and small and a nuisance to prepare but do add a pungent flavor to soups or use as potatoes and maybe mash with others. They usually need to have the outer skin taken off.

Horseradish   This is often overlooked as most people buy it in the jar. It has a pungent taste and is usually grated and mixed with cream or vinegar. Try cider vinegar.

Brassicas and Green Leafy Vegetables

- Buying and Storing- These do not keep well so always buy fresh and use as soon as possible.
- I find a lot of people have been put off eating some of the following vegetables because they had to eat them at school when they were boiled to death and stank! The best way to overcome this is to shred and eat them raw a completely different flavor and far more nutrients.

Broccoli There are purple sprouting and green varieties. Does not deserve to be boiled! It is best steamed or raw. Trim the larger stalk and add into soups. Trim the florets and sprinkle raw onto salads, the kids won't even notice it!

Cauliflower Steam or eat raw. Its great in salads; I actually like them in my vegetable curry after they have absorbed the flavor. It gives a different texture to the dish.

Cabbage There are quite a few varieties of cabbage. Try it shredded and eaten raw or lightly steamed. Mix with red cabbage for a colorful salad or stir fry and of course the "slaw".

Brussels Sprouts They are best after the first frost. Use the same as cabbage.

Kale This can be a little bitter if old so buy only young leaves and steam, stir fry or juice.

Spinach Spinach is a fabulous green vegetable, full of nutrients. Buy baby leaf and eat raw. The darker more mature greens only need a little light cooking. Wash and let the leaves stay wet; put a pan on the heat add the spinach; put the lid on for a few minutes and hey presto! You have a lovely dark-green vegetable dish.

Spinach apparently does not contain the iron that "Popeye" thought it did; Spinach contains oxalic acid which inhibits the absorption of iron and calcium; it is, however, a fantastic cancer-fighting antioxidant with about four times more beta carotene than broccoli. So it's well worth eating. If you have experienced a "bitter" taste it will be due to the kind of cooking, or the spinach is too old. Take the leaves away from any thick stems and put the stems into a vegetable stock for soup.

Swiss chard This is a member of the beet family, used in the same way as spinach and again does contain oxalic acid.

Spring Greens A leafy cabbage really, full flavor and yes, springtime is the best time to have this all new, green and lush. Shred and eat raw or lightly steamed.

Pumpkin and the Squash Family

- These arrive at different times of the year so there will always be a season for these versatile vegetables.
- Winter Squash tend to have a tough inedible skin with a dense and fibrous flesh and large seeds and can be used in both sweet and savory dishes. These are Acorn, Butternut and Pumpkin.
- Summer Squash are picked whilst young and the skins are tender, Patty pan, courgette/zucchini, marrows and cucumber.
- Always buy fresh; However Winter Squash will keep for several weeks if stored in a cool place.
- When peeling the winter squash take care as the outer skins are tough. Cut into chunks that you can deal with, discard the skin and seeds although you can roast the pumpkin seeds if you like after they have been dried.

Shoot Vegetables

Fennel — Florence fennel is closely related to the herb and spice of the same name. It has a similar texture to celery. The whole vegetable including the fronds are edible. It has quite a distinct aniseed flavor but cooking encourages sweetness. This vegetable can be sliced, chopped and included in salads, cut into quarters or eights, brushed with olive oil and roasted.

Asparagus — In the UK the season for this wonderful vegetable is late April till June although worldwide it is available at any time. A very therapeutic and visual vegetable simply cooked by poaching or roasted, which almost seems as shame but gives a different dimension. Drizzle with a little olive oil.

Chicory — Chicory is used in salads but needs to be combined with sweeter leaves as it can be slightly bitter in taste. You can steam or add to a stir fry.

Celery — A very medicinal vegetable, tangy in taste; if tasting bitter the celery is old. Can be eaten raw or braised but also can be added to soups or included in a vegetable stock.

Vegetable Fruits

Tomatoes — An all time favorite and very versatile fruit. Vine ripened in natural sunlight are best so eat seasonally. There are many varieties including cherry and plum. Sun dried tomatoes are so tasty added to salads, stir fry, a mezze and so on.

Aubergine/Eggplant A little understood and undervalued fruit. Most of us know it as an oval shape with a deep purple color. The smaller egg shaped variety is the one that has the name "eggplant" associated with it. It is a great addition to spicy casseroles and tomato based dishes such as ratatouille; roasted, stuffed and pureed into dips with lots of garlic. Don't buy huge ones as they will be tough and have more seeds. Do not buy them with damaged or wrinkly skins. They absorb a lot of oil so it is advisable not to fry them.

Chillies Members of the Capsicum family, chillies are widely used in Indian, Mexican and other spicy dishes. Unfortunately, most people use the dried powder (which is ok) but not quite like a fresh one. There are many varieties and shapes ranging in potency from very mild to very hot. The smaller ones tend to be the hottest, not by color. They can be red, green, yellow or orange depending on how they have ripened in the sun. Take care when preparing! I use rubber gloves to slice open and remove the seeds and white membrane as this is where the "hot" is at its most potent. Do not touch your face or eyes as they will sting like mad.

Peppers These come in a range of colors; the green ones are commonly less ripened which sometimes makes them harder to digest although they are so tasty and crisp. The other colors are generally sweeter. Great roasted, stuffed, raw, steamed lightly and then marinated in a flavored olive oil. Great addition to all tomato based recipes.

Avocado

Not understood as a health giving fruit because it is high in fat, but the fat is mono-saturated and therefore helps to lower cholesterol. Lots of protein and essential fatty acids makes this a very desirable food product. Slice in half and remove the stone, eat as it is or as a dressing or spoon in a tasty dip, cube into salads. Guacamole is a favorite dip which is in the recipe section

Pods and Seeds

Peas

Peas are a great favorite for both flavor and color. Pick as young and fresh as possible as they become starchy if left too long. Can be used in any way liked.

Broad Beans

Again, young and fresh are best. If they are larger you need to remove them from their pods and skins, a fiddly job but well worth it. Remove them from the outer pods and cook (blanch/boil) for a few minutes and the inner tender beans will pop out.

Green Beans

We have quite a variety of these, French, Runner, Dwarf and so on. Top and tail and steam are best, can be left to cool and eaten with salads or just eat raw.

Sweet Corn/Corn on the cob   Eat soon after picking; like peas they can be a bit starchy if left and the kernels get tough.

The Onion Family

Onions   A great variety of these and used in so many ways. They range in taste from sweet and juicy to a powerful and pungent taste. Shallots are delicious roasted with garlic. There are many culinary uses for onions, both raw and cooked.

Garlic   Garlic has a great many health benefits, starting with being anti-viral and anti-fungal. Whole garlic is sweet and great roasted or cooked in many dishes. Mincing, dicing or crushing the garlic gives off a more pungent taste. Only buy garlic bulbs if they are juicy and moist. They are semi-dried which prolongs the shelf life but discard if they have green shoots coming out or are dry. Summer or "wet" garlic looks a bit like a large spring onion and can be used in the same way as the dryer variety. Do not store in the fridge but keep in a cool dark place.

Leeks   Very versatile with a great taste, steamed, sauté, soup, shredded and stir fried. They are easy to clean, cut off the base and remove a layer of the outer skin, chop off the toughest of the green part whilst retaining some and then slice halfway through lengthways and wash. These often are gritty and this will wash them all the way through.

Mushrooms   There are many books on mushroom varieties, edible or non edible, Chinese to Portobello; Dried to fresh. It is well worth getting a book if you are interested in the benefits of these versatile food items. If you have an issue such as Candida or a respiratory problem, I do not recommend eating them as they are Fungi, grown in the damp and wet and throw off spores. See more on Candida or respiratory problems at: www.trishastewart.com

Salad Leaves

Red, dark green, light green, purple, peppery, sweet, bitter and so on. Such a variety these days which really jazz up the simplest salad or garnish. It is good to eat a raw salad with a cooked meal or as a starter as this encourages the digestive enzymes to flow.

Fruits

Fruit is the ultimate convenience food, washed and eaten on the go; juiced or used in a variety of salads, or bakes. Always buy firm fruits with no bruising or broken skins. They release fructose which is a natural sugar for energy.

Use homegrown fruit in season as naturally ripened fruits give off the best enzymes, vitamins and minerals, bioflavonoids and anti-oxidants.

Apples   Several varieties from Cox's Orange Pippin to the tart flavor of a Bramley. Used in both savory and sweet dishes alike; they are great for juicing, adding natural sweetness to a vegetable based juice.

Pears They are quite versatile in savory and sweet dishes. Raw, poached or baked. There are many varieties.

Apricots So much nicer fresh than dried, raw is best, sometimes they need to be cooked but this does give a lovely flavor.

Cherries Sweet are best eaten raw, Morello are sour and need cooking.

Plums Plums range in color from pale yellow to rich purple. Many varieties are sweet and tart. Can be cooked and pureed to make a sauce or fresh and raw in a fruit combo

Peaches and Nectarines These are very seasonal (in the UK) if you want them at their best. Eat raw with skin on preferably.

Citrus Varieties include oranges, lemons and limes, grapefruit, mandarins, and clementines to name a few.

These fruits need to be eaten when they are ripened in the sunlight and not stored in some container until shipped to wherever and then ripened in storage. The benefits and versatility of these fruits are worth waiting for and getting the best from. They are great sliced in hot water to drink, grated rind in dishes, dressings, sauces, whole fruit juiced and so on.

Berries and currants These are VERY seasonal in the UK but a great treat especially if you can pick from the hedgerows or home grown pickings. Choose from Strawberries, Raspberries, Blackberries, Blueberries, Gooseberries, Black currants, Red and White currants. Great fresh when picked, juiced, or pureed. Delightful!

Grapes, Melons, Dates and Figs

- Many varieties of grapes are used in wine making, juicing and eaten whole. Melons have high water content so they are great in the summer for quenching thirst. Eat aside from any other food as they digest very quickly and can inhibit the absorption and nutrients from other foods.
- Figs, such a delight when they are fresh, can be poached or baked. Dates eaten fresh are sweet and soft.

Tropical Fruit

- Pineapple and Papaya are great for the digestion as they contain the enzymes bromelain and papain. Also, they are great for juicing and fruit combos. Bananas are very starchy which is why they are so popular because they fill the hunger gap; mashed or blended makes a thick smoothie. For mangos check the skin for ripeness; a totally green skin is the sign of an unripe fruit.

Oils

- These provide us with essential fatty acids, vitamins and minerals.
- There are a wide variety of oils for cooking and for use in dressings.
- They are made from fruits, nuts and seeds and best extracted by slow mechanical means rather than being

put through a heat process which changes the properties. Choose first cold pressed, un-refined oils for flavor and nutrient value.

- Olive oil is, as it states, from olives usually grown in France, Greece, Italy or Spain. Generally, the hotter the climate, the more robust the oil is. It comes in Extra Virgin variety (which is premium oil) and best used for dressings or just drizzled over steamed vegetables; stirred into sauces etc. Virgin is also premium oil and is best used in the same way or mixed with lighter oils for cooking.
- Pure olive oil will be blended and refined, lighter in flavor and suitable for cooking, although over 100 degrees the properties change.

Corn	Corn oil is suitable for cooking.
Coconut	Coconut oil is very popular due to its ability to withstand higher temperature cooking. It is, however a saturated oil so not too much of it.
Safflower	Light all purpose oil, contains more polyunsaturated fat than any other type of oil, made from the seeds of the safflower. Keep for dressings.
Sunflower	Made from the seeds of the sunflower, good all purpose oil, not very strong in flavor. Good if mixed with olive or other oils for better flavor.
Soy	Useful for frying as it has a high smoking point and remains stable at high temperatures. Choose from non GM products.
Groundnut	Also know as peanut oil. Not much flavor.

Rapeseed	Very bland tasting all purpose oil. It is high in monosaturated fat.
Grape seed	Delicate flavor, made from seeds of the grapes left over from winemaking. Good all round use.
Sesame	The dark variety has a nutty aroma. It is used for flavoring marinades and in stir fry as it has a high smoking point. It is very strong in taste. The pale variety is from untoasted seeds and is lighter in flavor.
Walnut	Walnut oil is intensely flavored and delicious in salad dressings. Do not heat or cook as it is very expensive and far too good to waste.
Hazelnut	Fine and fragrant, do not waste this in cooking. Add to foods for flavor.
Almond	Almond oil is delicate and useful in both savory and sweet dishes and is often used as massage oil.

- There are many health benefits in these oils but do remember they are high in calories so use in moderation.
- Monosaturated oil particularly olive and rapeseed help to raise the good cholesterol HDL and contains vitamin E a natural anti-oxidant.
- Polyunsaturated fats provide us with the Omega 3 and 6
- All oils should be fresh and stored in a cool dark place.

Pasta

- I have great difficulty in advising the use of pasta; it is just wheat, water and sometimes egg depending on type of pasta. Buckwheat is gluten free so it has an advantage. I would not recommend using more than once a week and if you can use buckwheat, corn or rice pasta that would be preferable.

Noodles

- Same advice as for pasta.

Spices

- There are many spices, all with health benefits as well as adding a great taste to your food. It is always best to buy fresh and in small amounts; i.e. pods or seeds rather than ground as the flavor will be retained.

Allspice Small brown berries with a sweet flavor. They can be added to marinades or in oatcakes for a different flavor. It is sometimes added to curry for a sweeter taste. Grind before use. They are great for the digestion and for avoiding flatulence.

Cinnamon These come in sticks or a ready ground powder. The sticks can be used in sweet or savory dishes but remove the stick before serving. If stewing apple or pear put a stick in whilst simmering slowly. Cinnamon is great for cleansing and is anti-bacterial.

Caraway These little seeds have an aniseed flavor which works well with sweet or savory dishes. Can be used whole or slightly crushed. Nice added to potato, cabbage and carrots for a twist in flavor. Good for digestion and flatulence

Cardamom   The pods can be used whole or slightly crushed to release the full flavor. Works well in both savory and sweet dishes, often used in curry to bring a sweeter taste to the dish. Infused in hot rice or soy milk is a nice warm flavorsome drink. You can chew the seeds to freshen your breath. Calms digestion.

Cloves   These are mainly used in sweet dishes such as apple or pear. Use as cardamom but remove before serving. Long used as a cure for toothache for both its antiseptic and anaesthetic qualities.

Nutmeg   Nutmeg is used in sweet dishes, to add to porridge but can also work well to liven up savory sauces. Buy the whole fruit and grate as required. Good for digestion.

Cayenne   Cayenne is a fiery spice which adds color and heat but not too much in the way of taste. It is from the capsicum family so you will be familiar with chillies and peppers. It is a digestive stimulant so anyone with a sensitive digestion should avoid this as it can aggravate the stomach.

Chillies   I have already said earlier that fresh are best so use a very little amount of the powder. Be careful if your digestive system is sensitive.

Coriander   Coriander/cilantro, along with cumin rate highly in curry making. The seeds have a different flavor than the fresh leaves. Grind the seeds as required for a quality flavor. Good for digestion.

Cumin Cumin is used in curry making but also works well with tomato based dishes. It has a slightly bitter taste. Use whole seeds and grind. Dry frying for 60 seconds enhances the flavor.

Fenugreek Another popular spice used in curry making. A bitter taste, seeds are hard to grind. Good for digestion and cleansing.

Ginger Where possible always use the ginger root as the flavor is far more satisfying than the powder. This is so versatile- it can be used in soups, curries, and stir fry; marinades, juicing and added to hot water. It is great for the digestion and the immune system. The best way to handle this is to peel the root and freeze, when you need to grate it pull it out of the freezer and grate. Or just peel and slice.

Lemon Grass This comes in a long fibrous stalk, it has a citrus flavor and used in Thai cooking. It adds a lovely flavor when used with coconut. Remove the woody outer layer, remove the root and crush or chop finely.

Galangal Looks like ginger root. Prepare and use in the same way as ginger.

Paprika Milder than Cayenne, but still be aware if you have digestive problems.

Saffron Very expensive if you buy a quality product but you only need a small amount. Adds a bitter sweet taste but often is used because it adds a lovely color to rice or other dishes. Good for calming the digestive system.

| **Turmeric** | Used as an alternative to Saffron, it adds an earthy or peppery taste as well as an interesting yellow to rice or other dishes. It has anti-bacterial and anti-fungal properties. |

| **Vanilla** | I recommend using this to flavor porridge but only buy the pod which you can infuse and remove to be used again or pure essence. You can also use it with fruits, soy or rice milk drinks. |

Herbs

There are many herbs that can be found growing as nature intended and for us to collect and use for the therapeutic values but most of us manage to grow some in the garden on a window ledge or buy them from the local shops or farms.

I will name but a few here just to give you an idea on why to use them.

Bay Leaf (sweet laurel) A spicy, aromatic herb and is used in cooking for soups, casseroles, bouquet garni. To make it even more worthwhile use its benefits to aid digestion, reduce flatulence and (is also known) to treat influenza and bronchitis. An infusion of the crushed berries acts like a diuretic and is anti-rheumatic. Fresh is milder than dried but both are excellent in cooking.

Basil (sweet)   The Italian ingredient for pesto or the French for Provencal soupe au pisto.   It has a wonderful aroma. Freshly shred on tomatoes or in tomato soup, lovely flavor on salads. It is lovely used on any foods.   Fresh is definitely best.

Therapeutic uses include sedative and anti-spasmodic. It is also a digestive aid, helpful in nervous disorders and headaches, vertigo and colic in children. Other uses have been the fresh juice from the leaves poured into the ears is said to ease inflammation; and as an infusion, a gargle for thrush.

Chives   A lovely summer addition to salads, soups, cream or cheeze (vegan). Pretty garnish with its lovely green spiky leaves.

Dill   Is best used raw with any salad or vegetable. Dill leaves soaked in water overnight and used as a drink helps to calm the stomach.

Marjoram   Blends well with Thyme and Basil for sauces and vegetable casseroles. Medicinal use as a sedative; only small doses should be taken. Also soothes the digestive system and helps with the endocrine (hormonal) system. Its antiseptic values are used in tonsillitis, colds and respiratory problems. Compresses or lotions help with wound healing, also used in herb pillows for its relaxing and calming effects.

Mint   A well know herb. As with most herbs there are several varieties but generally speaking mint is used as an antiseptic, mouth wash, digestive aid, made into teas, sauces and jellies.

Parsley   The garnish everyone leaves on their plate!!! There are several varieties. Used to combat the smell of garlic on your breath, parsley juice is also a good mosquito repellent; a mild laxative and diuretic. It is used in cooking as part of a bouquet garni, salads, soups, casseroles. It is rich in Vitamin C, iron, magnesium and other vitamins and minerals.

Rosemary   Was also a symbol of friendship, love and fidelity. Its culinary uses are mainly soups and stews. This herb is also a stimulant and can be a useful tonic for invalids, depressives.

Sage   Several varieties and widely used in cooking stews, sprinkled on roasted vegetables. Its medicinal values are hormonal (PMS, menopause), soothing pain, nervous system regulator and stimulates circulation.

Tarragon   Several varieties widely used in cooking sauces, marinades and stuffing. Medicinally used as a digestive aid,

Thyme   There are several varieties. It is a good tonic and digestive aid; It helps with circulation, coughs and colds and is of hormonal benefit (regulating hormones). It is used widely in cooking as part of a bouquet garni; in soups, stews and vegetable dishes.

Coriander   (Green plant) widely used in salads and curries, the flavor of the fresh leaf and the seeds are quite different. Use fresh towards the end of the cooking and seeds at the beginning. Its medicinal purposes are thought to help eliminate toxic waste such as metals from the body (mercury (tooth fillings), cadmium and lead.

- There are many more herbs but as you can see they are very useful as part of your meal as most of them aid digestion. They help to produce enzymes and are enriched with vitamins and minerals.
- When trying to ease off salt and cut out junk food etc. the one thing people say they miss is the taste Ugh!! But of course those foods are so strong in salt, msg and other food additives which is what people are tasting- not real food. So adding herbs both fresh and dried makes lots of difference to the taste.
- Seaweeds are also great substitutes for salt, they have salt naturally occurring and a strip of Kombu in a soup makes all the difference.

Natural Sweetner

Agave Nectar (syrup)

- To produce agave nectar, juice is expressed from the core of the agave tree, called the *piña*. The juice is filtered, and then heated, to hydrolyze carbohydrates into sugars.
- Agave nectars are sold in light, amber, dark, and raw varieties. Light agave nectar has a mild, almost neutral flavor, and is a great choice for use in delicate tasting deserts, baked goods, sauces, and beverages. Amber agave nectar has a medium-intensity caramel flavor, and is suitable for many desserts, as well as sauces and savory dishes. Dark agave nectar has stronger almost caramel taste to flavor desserts. Raw agave nectar also

has a mild, neutral taste. It is produced at temperatures below 118 degrees F to protect the natural enzymes, so this variety is a perfect sweetener for raw food and the health conscious.

- Use one third of what would normally be used if using refined sugar.
- It must not be forgotten though; this is a sugar and will be high in calories and could cause a rapid rise in blood sugar levels - so diabetics and people with sugar handling problems must be aware.

Allergies and Intolerances

There may be people reading this book who are saying, I can't eat this or that because I have a food allergy.

A true food allergy will cause an immunologic reaction. The Immune system is over-stimulated by a certain food or allergen and attacks the body. The body will manufacture immunoglobulin E (IgE) antibodies which will react to the food or allergen and cause the immune system to release histamines and other chemicals causing an "allergic" response. Symptoms can be as little as bloating, diarrhea, constipation, to skin rashes, swelling of the throat, face tongue to loss of consciousness and in fact death.

Most people I see in my clinic do NOT have food allergies; they have food intolerances due to poor digestive function.

Food intolerance is a condition where adverse effects occur after eating a particular food, combination of foods or an ingredient in a food. These could be headaches, nausea, bloating, diarrhea, skin irritation, blocked sinuses, tiredness etc. and can occur at anytime from eating to 72 hours so it is really hard to detect which particular food or combination of foods that has been eaten that has caused the symptom.

This is not necessarily an immune response it is due to a compromised digestive system, often associated with candida and parasites, too much of one particular food which will cause the system to become compromised. However, there is a mass of lymphoid tissue in the gut which, if under constant attack will get weakened and will react to foods that may otherwise be harmless.

In my clinic I see these daily; chronic fatigue, fibromyalgia, tired all the time; headaches/migraine, IBS, colitis, period pain, menopausal symptoms, eczema, asthma, psoriases and so on, all can be attributed to a compromised gut and of course stress can create a worsening effect.

Depending on severity of condition, length of time suffered, a change of diet, supplementation and healing remedies are all that is needed to restore good health and vitality.

Cookware

Pots, pans and other cookware are made from a variety of materials. These materials can enter the food that we cook in them. Most of the time, this is harmless. However, care should be taken with some materials.

Aluminum

The perils of aluminum pans have been well known for some time. There is already far too much of this metal in the food chain and in bodywash, shampoo, toothpaste and other products. Aluminum has been associated with Alzheimer's disease but there is no definite proof as yet. The World Health Organization estimates that adults can consume more than 50 milligrams of aluminum daily without harm? No thanks is what I say.

As with any metal cookware there will be a certain amount that will leach into foods, particularly those foods such as leafy vegetables, citrus and tomatoes. The problem with aluminum is that it dissolves most easily from worn or pitted pots and pans.

Anodized Aluminum Cookware

There is a slight improvement using this type of cookware as the surface is harder and non scratch therefore reducing the amount or the possibility of leaching into foods.

Copper

The cookware of the professionals as the heat is evenly distributed. Copper in small amounts is good for us but like anything a large amount can be toxic and also coming from a pan, what else may be in this? Copper pans often come with a stainless steel cooking surface. Probably best left as a decoration over the fireplace.

Stainless Steel and Iron Cookware

Stainless steel and Iron cookware are probably the safest depending on any other metal that is mixed with it during the manufacturing process.

Nickel and Chromium are probably the two metals that may leach out of this cookware in small quantities and relatively harmless but remember the "totting up" system I use with foods, the same applies so cut down on processed foods and highly available body and hair products and cleaning materials.

Ceramic

Ceramic cookware is glazed; similar glazes are applied to metals to make enamelware. These glazes, a form of glass, resist wear and corrosion.

The problem here is the use of pigments such as lead and cadmium in making the glaze and the chemicals involved.

Glass

This material should be harmless unless of course there are chemicals that go into the glazing. The problem is heating to high temperatures.

Plastics

For cooking and storing food are fine as long as there is no heat placed upon them; so using in a microwave could prove to be harmful. Using plastic containers and wrap for anything other than their original purpose can cause health problems. Wrapping foods in plastic cling film again is ok but do not add heat because this will release chemicals that can harm us. Plastic is known to be estrogenic and therefore may be the cause of infertility in men.

Non-stick

There has been lots of news on non-stick coatings which are applied to metal pans to prevent food from sticking and help reduce the amount of oil needed. The coating is likely to be carcinogenic, there are several independent studies performed on rats which of course like all these studies is appalling. The product widely used in the coating is Perfluorooctanoic and its salts known as PFOA. The biggest problem is the poisonous fumes from the coating when the pans are heated and of course using old chipped and worn ones.

So what can you do? You have to cook and store foods.

Minimize your risks by the following:

- It would be a good idea to get rid of all aluminum cookware. If you decide not to, do not store cooked foods in these pans.
- Get rid of all cookware that is chipped, flaking or not at its best.
- Beware of nickel if you are allergic or have an intolerance to it as some people do when touching this metal.

- Do not store any citrus fruits, green leafy vegetables or tomato based meals in any metal pan.
- Do not heat plastic bowls or cling film.
- If using ceramic beware of cheap products as they may contain chemicals in the manufacture and glazing.

Sprouting

The easiest way to explain this is you can sprout nuts, seeds and pulses in the same way you used to grow mustard and cress as kids.

Nuts   If you are going to make cheeze, nut butter or cream, soak them. For sprouting they will need 24 hours soaking (less for softer nuts like cashews, pecans and walnuts) and will then germinate in around 1-2 days. Half a cup of nuts will yield around three quarters of a cup of sprouted nuts. Rinse am and pm, do not allow them to dry out. Put in the refrigerator which will stunt their growth if you are not quite ready for them.

Seeds   If you are making cheeze, nut butter, milk or cream you need only soak for 12 - 24 hours. For sprouting, (except alfalfa), most will take 1-3 days and they need rinsing twice daily too. A quarter cup of seeds will make around half to one cup of sprouts. To retard their growth, put in the refrigerator. Alfalfa requires a longer harvesting time, 6 days or more, they yield a massive harvest from just a quarter of a cup, they will fill a gallon container. Others such as clover, radish, chive, onion and garlic too will require a big container to grow in.

Beans (pulses) and Legumes (lentils and peas)

The soaking time for these is 24 hours. These will triple in volume once sprouted and take around 2-4 days before you can harvest them. They are great blended into soups or raw on salads and main dishes.

Grains   Buckwheat, kamut, rye all need around 8 hours soaking and will be ready to harvest in 1-2 days.

Equipment needed:

A sprout bag or a screw top jar, a colander or tiered sprouting trays

Some of the most popular ones to sprout:

- Alfalfa
- Clover
- Fenugreek
- Chives
- Onion
- Garlic
- Broccoli and Cabbage
- Radish
- Mustard
- Wheat grass
- Sunflower seeds
- Flax seeds
- Pumpkin Seeds
- Peas
- Quinoa (any grains will sprout)
- Lentils
- Beans (mung, adzuki, chick pea, turtle and so on)
- Nuts (almond, cashew, pecans, walnuts, brazils, macadamias)

Why sprout?

- Easier on digestion due to these being young plants (once sprouted) the enzymes are available to help with digestion
- More nutritious, being young plants they are picked/harvested at their prime giving the body a mass of vitamins, minerals, proteins, enzymes, bioflavonoids.
- Economical cheap to buy, cheap to grow, a few seeds go a long way,
- Completely organic (providing one has purchased organic seeds)
- You can eat these at any time of the year,
- Totally fresh as they are grown and harvested quickly
- Versatile as you can add them to salads, soups, stir fry, juices. They will add a new dimension to the look and taste of your foods.

How to sprout

- Get your container cleaned and ready
- Soak the seeds or whatever you are going to sprout overnight
- Drain and rinse in the morning
- Place in the container you are going to grow them in and rinse again, preferably with a spray attachment.
- Cover with the plastic or the lid to the container you are using or make a tunnel over the seed tray
- Twice daily rinsing am and pm

Gadgets

There will be plenty of time saving gadgets on the market so for you "gadget" people, go get them as they may be time saving but I still like some of the old ways of doing things. Here are a few that may interest you and prove to be really helpful, some you cannot do without.

Blender

> I think an absolute must, you will notice in these recipes how many times it is used. Buy the best quality you can as you will be using it for lots of things and the motors burn out quickly in the cheaper ones.

Food Processor

> Again, something you will use time and time again, you will find that a good one will blend as well so this gets rid of the blender. Get one that grinds chops, grates, shreds, and blends.

Hand Mixer/Stick Blender

> These are great little whizzers that you can put straight into the pot of soup or large jug and whizz up as much as you want. Again, well worth buying one as it saves on washing up your blender or processor; only one piece to wash!

Juicer

> This is a commitment to juicing. Buy something like a Green Star" or "Champion" as these will give you the best juice ever plus it will make your nut butters, cream, cheeze, ice creams and also will juice

wheatgrass. They are expensive but well worth it if you are going to use it. The cheaper ones which have the blades create too much heat and begin to destroy the enzymes.

Citrus Juicer

This is a great, simple little gadget which presses really well. Well worth having one.

Knives

Although in a lot of cases you can tear vegetables and salads a good sharp knife is invaluable. Invest in a good quality stainless steel paring knife (small), serrated knife and a large knife for big vegetables and if you are a "dab hand" with your knife you will use it to slice up onions and other vegetables as you see the chef's do on TV!

Electric Knife Sharpener

A handy gadget if you have invested in good quality knives. Beware! When you have these knives in tip top condition they will slice a finger off no problem – do not let the kids use them, please.

Mandolin

This is a hand held slicer, shredder or grater; a cheap and cheerful little tool and very handy especially if you are only preparing for yourself.

Salad Spinner

A really good and very small investment dries your leaves in record time.

Mesh Bags or Muslin Cloths

Good for straining nut milk or yogurt when making Tsatziki.

Nut Grinder or Seed Mill

You may get one of these with your blender but there are some good ones for just doing that job, again, time saved on washing a huge blender or processor.

Pestle and Mortar

Old fashioned but I love these, they look nice left out on the kitchen top too. Just put your salt, herbs, spices, garlic or whatever you want to pulverize and grind away. They are easy to wash and have no mechanical parts.

Pots and Pans

You will see I have dedicated a section to just pans. You will need a variety of pots; glass or ceramic, whatever you like that will withstand oven temperatures. Also some nice serving dishes; try to combine both to save on washing up.

Sprouting Equipment

A simple colander will do, or a sprouting bag, jar, or those fancy tiered trays. If it can sprout, it will grow anywhere as long as watered twice daily. See section on sprouting.

Steamer

You can get a stand-alone electric one or a stainless steel one that sits on a pan of simmering water. These are useful to lightly cook all the side vegetables you will be having.

Garlic Press

Cheap and easy to use, will mince very finely and useful in some recipes where you don't want slices or chopped garlic.

Shopping List

Not complete as you will need to choose what actual ingredients will work for you - but this is a great place to start!

Store Cupboard Ingredients

Grains Porridge oats, Millet, Quinoa *(pronounced "keen wa")*, Buckwheat, Bulghur Wheat, Wholegrain rice, Wild Rice, Cornflour , Rice Flour, Potato Flour, Soya Flour, Pure Baking Powder

Legumes Lentils, (green, red, brown, puy), Peanuts

Beans/Pulses Chick Peas, Mung, Black Turtle, Black eyed, Kidney, Flageolot, Haricot, Pinto, Butter, Borlotti, Cannellini.

Pasta Rice Noodles, Rice Pasta or Corn Pasta

Miscellaneous

- Sun dried tomato paste, Tomato paste, Passata, Tamarind pulp, Yeast free stock - Marigold Swiss Boullion is good, low salt
- Carob powder or Cacao nibs
- Vanilla beans or Pure essence, Pure almond essence
- Pure Maple Syrup, Agave nectar, Honey (for non vegans)
- Dried fruits (ensure sulphur free)

- Seaweeds - I have only used Hiijiki in this book, but if you want to put Kombu into a soup to add to the flavor of the stock, don't forget to buy it.
- Shitake and Porcini dried mushrooms
- Dried red chillies
- Tamari Sauce, Balsamic Vinegar, Apple Cider Vinegar, Tahini, Mirin, rice wine. Pure Tabasco and Jalapeno sauce
- Tinned Tomatoes and pulses/beans for emergency use, check no sugar/salt.
- Black pepper, pure sea salt, mustard powder/seeds
- Rice milk, Soya milk, Coconut milk or Cream

Oil   Extra Virgin Olive Oil, Sesame Oil, Walnut Oil, Coconut oil,

Herbs (dried) Basil, Thyme, Sage, Rosemary, Bay leaf, Marjoram, Tarragon, Coriander (leaf), oregano

Spices (Use seeds where possible and grind for freshness)

- Sweet paprika, Cayenne pepper, Black peppercorns, White peppercorns, Celery seed, Coriander seed, Cinnamon sticks, Nutmeg, Chilli powder, Garam masala, Cumin, Fenugreek, Fennel, Tumeric, Saffron, Poppy seed, Star Anise, Cloves, Curry leaves,Kaffir Lime Leaves, Lemon Grass (dried),

Seeds   sunflower, pumpkin, sesame, hemp, flax/linseeds

Nuts   Cashews, brazils, macadamia, hazelnuts, walnuts, almonds, pecans

Seed	Sesame, Sunflower, Pumpkin, Flax/linseed, Poppy

To Sprout

- Check sprouting in the book on page 170 as there are many to choose from

Fresh Ingredients, just a few ideas, buy what is in season and of course what you fancy

Fresh vegetables/salads

- Carrots, swede, turnips, parsnip, kohlrabi, sweet potato, squash/pumpkin, beetroot, onions, garlic, scallions, shallots, artichokes, cabbage red/green/white, spinach, kale, broccoli, brussell sprouts, cauliflower, asparagus. Swiss chard, green beans. Various herb leaves, lettuce, cucumber, courgette (zucchini), peppers, celery, aubergine/eggplant.

Miscellaneous

- Fresh chilies, ginger, garlic
- Tofu – smoked, plain, herbed (not strictly fresh – found in the chiller cabinet)

Fruit

- Apples, Pears, Apricots, Cherries, Plums, Peaches, Nectarines, Oranges, Grapefruit, Lemons and Limes, Mandarins, Berries of all kinds, Grapes, Melons, Dates, Figs, Pineapple, Papaya, Bananas, Mango.

Conversion Table

Cup	Oz	Grams	tbsp.	tsp.	Fl. Oz.	ml
1/16	1/2	14	1	3	1/2	15
1/8	1	28	2	6	1	30
3/16	1-1/2	43	3	9	1-1/2	44
1/4	2	57	4	12	2	59
5/16	2-1/2	71	5	15	2-1/2	74
3/8	3	85	6	18	3	89
7/16	3-1/2	99	7	21	3-1/2	104
1/2	4	113	8	24	4	118
9/16	4-1/2	128	9	27	4-1/2	133
5/8	5	142	10	30	5	148
11/16	5-1/2	156	11	33	5-1/2	163
3/4	6	170	12	36	6	177
13/16	6-1/2	184	13	39	6-1/2	192
7/8	7	199	14	42	7	207
15/16	7-1/2	213	15	45	7-1/2	222
1	8	227	16	48	8	237
1-1/16	8-1/2	241	17	51	8-1/2	251
1-1/8	9	255	18	54	9	266
1-3/16	9-1/2	269	19	57	9-1/2	281
1-1/4	10	284	20	60	10	296

Trisha Stewart

> *We are indeed much more than what we eat, but what we eat can nevertheless help us to be much more than what we are.*

Adelle Davis *(1904 - 1974)*

180